THE AFRICAN-AMERICAN GUIDE TO

Living Well with Diabetes

The African-American Guide to

Living Well with Diabetes

Constance Brown-Riggs,
MSEd, RD, CDE, CDN,

with Tamara Jeffries

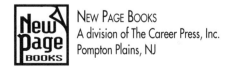

NEW PAGE BOOKS
A division of The Career Press, Inc.
Pompton Plains, NJ

THE AFRICAN AMERICAN GUIDE TO LIVING WELL WITH DIABETES
EDITED BY KATE HENCHES
TYPESET BY EILEEN MUNSON
Cover design by Dutton & Sherman Design
Printed in the U.S.A. by Courier

To order this title, please call toll-free 1-800-CAREER-1 (NJ and Canada: 201-848-0310) to order using VISA or MasterCard, or for further information on books from Career Press.

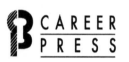

The Career Press, Inc., 220 West Parkway, Unit 12,
Pompton Plains, NJ 07444
www.careerpress.com
www.newpagebooks.com

Library of Congress Cataloging-in-Publication Data
Brown-Riggs, Constance.
  The African American guide to living well with diabetes / by Constance Brown-Riggs ; with Tamara Jeffries.
     p. cm.
  Includes bibliographical references and index.
  ISBN 978-1-60163-115-2 -- ISBN 978-1-60163-728-4 (ebook) 1. Diabetes. 2. African Americans--Diseases. 3. Diabetes--Diet therapy. 4. Diabetes--Diet therapy--Recipes. 5. Diabetes--Exercise therapy. I. Jeffries, Tamara. II. Title.

  RC662.B748 2010
  616.4'62008996073--dc22

                                                                    2010008936

This book is dedicated to my mother,
Murlie Gatling,
who taught me
"nothing beats a failure but a try;"
my father,
James Gatling,
who encouraged me to always
"cross that bridge when you get to it;"
and my husband,
Lawrence,
for his incredible patience and support.
—C.B.R.

In memory of my grandmother,
Fannie Sutherlin Gwynn,
who managed her diabetes with care.
And to my aunts and uncles who follow in her footsteps.
—T.J.

Acknowledgments

This book would not have been possible without the encouragement and support of so many wonderfully talented people. My heartfelt thanks to:

My "less-melanated soul sister," Marlisa Brown for bringing my manuscript to the attention of her agent, Stephany Evans. And to Stephany, now my agent, who was able to look past the rough edges of my manuscript and envision a great book.

Jodi Wright, for her comprehensive research and assistance in completing the nutritional analysis of the recipes.

Those who contributed the delicious recipes: Chef Josué Merced Reyes, Chef Marc Anthony Bynum, Leslene Gordon, Fabienne Volel, and Jessica Jones. And my husband, Lawrence, for cooking and tasting recipes and developing a few of his own culinary delights.

My brother Rev. Marvin G. Gatling for his contribution to and spiritual guidance on the For Your Spirit sections.

Tamara Jeffries, an incredibly gifted and talented writer and editor who was able to make my work readable and understandable. Thank you for saying yes when it would have been easier to say no.

Micheal Pye and the decision-makers at New Page Books, who understood my vision and saw the importance of such a book.

And a big hug for "Grandma's love joy," Sadaijah Tamir Andrews. Now grandma will spend more time with you.

Contents

INTRODUCTION:
ONE DAY AT A TIME

On any given Sunday morning in African-American congregations across the nation, choirs and church folk sing the plaintive refrain to the popular gospel song, "One Day at a Time."

As with so many gospel songs, this one was written as a result of struggle and adversity. The writer, Marijohn Wilkin, was at a very low point in her life when she penned the words to the now-classic song in 1980. Though she'd been a successful writer, she suffered from depression and alcoholism and had become suicidal after the breakup of three marriages. As she began to turn her life around, the words to the song became a source of relief and inspiration for her, as it has been for many who sing or listen to and reflect on the words.

It may seem odd to open a book about diabetes with a gospel hymn, but it makes sense in that, though it may not have been Wilkin's intention, the words of "One Day at a Time" provide inspiration that is as appropriate for someone facing a health challenge as it is for someone dealing with a spiritual crisis. In fact, when you are diagnosed with a chronic disease for which there is no immediate cure—a disease like diabetes—the challenge can be just as much mental and spiritual as it is physical.

Think about it. Diabetes is sometimes called the silent disease because, unless it's already out of control, it isn't particularly painful or uncomfortable or physically debilitating. But it is something that you have to cope with every day. You must monitor your blood sugar, take your medicine or, perhaps, inject yourself with insulin. You have to carefully attend to what you eat, watching sugar and counting carbohydrates ("carbs"). You need to get more exercise; but you have to make sure you don't injure your feet. And you have to stay on top of all of that every day. Because once you have it, the disease is part your life. When you get up in the morning you have diabetes; when you go to bed at night you still have diabetes.

The daily-ness of chronic disease can leave you feeling overwhelmed, powerless, and exhausted. And on some days, you may find that those feelings are more challenging than the physical symptoms. Those are the days when you have to search for inspiration, for discipline, for hope. It's on those days that the words in Marijohn Wilkins' song will seem so relevant: *Teach me today to do all the things that I have to do.*

Your physical diagnosis may require certain care, but you have to be in the right frame of mind with the right intention of spirit to care for yourself properly, consistently, and wisely.

Why the "Mental" Matters

If you're reading this book, you or someone you care about has been diagnosed with diabetes. That means a doctor has already told you what you need to do to take care of yourself. Depending on your understanding, your doc's communication skills and the specifics of your case (everybody's diagnosis is different) you may have come away with some pretty straight-forward instruction. *I can handle this,* you think. And you can.

But one day you'll have a particularly difficult day at work, and you'll come home exhausted. Though you know exercise is good for you and helps you keep your sugar low, you just won't feel up to going out for a jog or stopping at the gym.

Or maybe you'll find yourself a little stressed out by some family drama. If there's one thing that sooths your nerves, it's a little bit of chocolate-chip ice cream—and you just happen to have some in the freezer, so you take out the carton and a spoon and enjoy a sweet, creamy frozen dinner.

Then Thanksgiving will come around, a time when your whole family gathers for a mini family reunion. After you feast on Uncle Bud's deep-fried turkey, candied yams, macaroni and cheese, collard greens with ham hocks, good old-fashion cornbread, and three kinds of cake, you'll sit around the table talking, laughing, reminiscing—and absentmindedly nibbling at the leftovers. Time will fly by and you will have forgotten all about checking your blood sugar.

Christmas will come with gifts and goodies. It will be too cold to jog in January. April 15 will roll around and you'll crunch away tax-time stress with bags of chips. You'll nibble too many rich hors d'oeuvres at a wedding, or accept too thick a slice of birthday cake at a party. You'll forget your glucose monitor when you go on vacation. And day-by-day, decision-by-decision, you'll be handling your diabetes, alright. But you won't be handling it well. And before you know it, your diabetes will be handling you.

You heard the doctor. You know you should watch your diet, get daily exercise, and monitor your sugar. And you have the best intentions. But unless you are extremely disciplined and dedicated to taking care of yourself, there are going to be times when your mental state or your emotional life will interfere with doing what you know your body needs. In fact, even the most conscientious patient will have lapses. We're only human, after all.

But because you're human—and you happen to be a human with a chronic condition—you have to do everything you can to support yourself in taking care of your diabetes. That's why, if you want to live long and live well with diabetes, you can't just address it as a physical condition. You have to take a mind, body, and spirit approach. That is what this book is designed to help you do.

All You Need

The African-American Guide to Living Well with Diabetes is the book that will give you all the information you need to manage your condition for the long haul. And I know a lot of books may say that. And many of them out there will give you lots of information on drugs, diet, and exercise. But the book you're holding does two things that the others won't.

First, it's not written for just anybody. It's written for "us"—because we need and deserve something that speaks to our unique relationship with diabetes. Some research indicates that we're just genetically more prone to the disease—and the numbers seem to bear that out. Of the almost 24 million people who are diagnosed with diabetes, four million are African-Americans. A fourth of Black women older than age 55 have it; a quarter of all Black folks between the ages of 65 and 74 do too. And we suffer greater consequences from the long-term complications of diabetes than our less-melanated brothers and sisters.

Not only are we more likely to have it, but we manage it differently than other people might. Our approach to exercise, our eating habits, and our relationships with doctors—all of that has an impact on how we approach our health conditions. And all of that was taken into consideration as this book was being written.

The second unique thing about this book is that it incorporates what is perhaps the most important part of our culture: our spirituality. This book does not assume we all belong to the same religion. Among us are Baptists, Buddhists, Baha'i, Muslims, Methodists, and even a Mormon or two. But, as a whole, we tend to be a community of believers—and the spirituality that infuses our lives has an impact on how we feel about physical affliction, healing, and the relationship between faith and medicine. Your beliefs will have an overt or subtle influence on how you cope with your condition, so we address your spiritual health right along with all the physical aspects of your condition. In fact, each chapter closes with a passage called "For Your Spirit," an inspirational, encouraging message that brings home the connection between what's going on in your body and what's happening in your soul.

Because people of color tend to be people of faith, many of us approach our health challenges as a test of our spiritual beliefs. That can be a good thing. Even some folks in the medical community are coming around to the idea that prayer, meditation, affirmation, and belief in a Higher Power can help keep us healthier and aid us in overcoming illness. Many people who believe that you can use your spirituality to bring blessings into your life or push unwanted events away, use the phrase "don't claim it" to mentally dismiss an illness. The phrase is designed to help us fortify ourselves mentally and spiritually when we are fighting disease. But when we take "don't claim it" to mean "ignore it"—and fail to seek the care we need—we put at risk the very temple created to house our spirit. We don't want to take it there. This book reclaims "don't claim it" as a statement of encouragement that you can use as armor as you cope with the challenges of living with diabetes. It's an affirmation that you can overcome the disease—if you use all of the tools that Spirit has provided.

What's Inside

In the chapters that follow you will get a comprehensive definition and description of diabetes in all its forms, as well as the treatments and medications that are available to help you manage the disease and cope with (if not avoid) the complications that can accompany it. Because most African-Americans who are diagnosed with diabetes will have type 2, known as adult-onset diabetes, most of the information in this book will focus on that type. But all types of diabetes—type 1 (so-called juvenile diabetes) and type 2—require similar care. The key to living well with *any* kind of diabetes is to eat well, exercise, take insulin or oral medications if they're prescribed and work closely with your healthcare provider. We'll introduce you to the team of doctors, specialists, and other caregivers who are available to guide your care—and give you tips on how to communicate with them so that you're all working together for the best benefit of your health.

Of course we'll devote a lot of space in this book to talking about what you can and can't eat. (Short version: You can eat pretty much anything you want. It's all in how you do it.) In several chapters, we will address the basics of good nutrition, building a diabetes-specific food pyramid, interpreting food labels, counting carbohydrates, and monitoring and managing your blood-sugar levels.

Because a healthy weight and good fitness level are key to living well with diabetes, we'll spend some time talking about diets—the healthy ones that work, the alternative ones that may have some benefits, and the fad diets that may do more harm than good. The chapter on fitness will help you design an exercise routine that will not only help you lose weight—an important part of managing diabetes—but will keep you motivated and mentally sharp for the long haul.

You'll learn ways to address denial and the other complex emotions that often come along with a diabetes diagnosis, and how to develop the habits—discipline, a positive attitude, good follow-through—that you'll need to overcome the mental blocks to taking the best possible care of yourself.

No two diabetes patients have the same situation, so part of your challenge will be to develop a self-care program that works for you. That's why each chapter includes charts and worksheets that will help you do things like develop your own meal plan, organize a personal fitness program, manage your glucose levels, keep track of relevant information, and even manage your moods. And, though we hope you will read each page with as much care as it was written, we know you'll sometimes need info in a hurry, so each chapter concludes with a Power Points section—a quick summary of the most important take-away points in the chapter.

In the back of the book you will find three appendices: The first is a two-week sample menu chock full of Caribbean and traditional Southern meal-time favorites—with carb counts and nutrient totals conveniently included. Appendix B provides select recipes from the sample menus— each analyzed for nutrient totals. And Appendix C is a list of the carb counts of more than 100 traditional foods from the American South and Caribbean designed to help you successfully incorporate your favorite fare into your daily meal planning.

Ultimately, this book covers absolutely every aspect of living with diabetes. It will become your self-care bible. And a bible is exactly what you will need to live well with diabetes—body, mind, and soul.

Living well with diabetes is a life-long process. Your goal is to maintain good health each day of your life, "one day at a time." The beginning of the familiar song reminds us, *"I'm only human. I'm just a woman."* No one is perfect and diabetes by its very nature is unpredictable, so there will be days when you've done everything "right" and your blood sugar will still be higher than expected. Don't be discouraged. "Yesterday's gone," as the song says. Tomorrow is an opportunity to start fresh. Take this book along with you as you travel the road to living well with diabetes.

1 Diabetes: What It Is, What It Does

Diabetes affects our pancreas and kidneys, but it can also cause problems with our feet and limbs. It runs in families, but you won't necessarily get it just because your mother did. We call it sugar, but if you have it, it's anything but sweet. It's one of the most familiar diseases in our community—and yet myths about diabetes abound. So what is diabetes really?

Here's the short version: You'll be diagnosed with diabetes if your blood-glucose level—the sugar in your blood—is consistently above normal. Having high blood sugar is a sign that your body isn't making enough insulin or using insulin properly. Insulin is the hormone that helps move that glucose into your cells to be used as energy. But if insulin isn't doing its job, glucose will just stay in the bloodstream, eventually causing trouble with the way your internal organs function.

Perhaps a better way to describe what diabetes is, is to explain how the body works when you *don't* have it.

Diabetes Defined

After you eat—especially if you're eating carbohydrate-rich foods such as bread, cereal, fruit, and milk—the body changes your meal into the form of sugar called glucose. As the food moves into the intestines, that glucose is absorbed into the blood stream. In the intestines, "helper hormones" alert the pancreas to release insulin, a hormone that takes the glucose out of the blood stream and helps it to enter the cells of the body, where it can be stored or used as a source of energy. Insulin not only regulates sugar, it also affects how the body uses fat and protein from the food you eat: It lets fat enter the cells to be stored or used as energy much in the same way that glucose is used. It also helps make protein available to repair cells of your organs and muscles.

That's when everything is going according to plan. When you have diabetes, there's a glitch somewhere in the system. Either your body does not make enough insulin or insulin isn't used properly, or you don't have enough of the "helper hormones" to stimulate the release of insulin from the pancreas. The end result is a buildup of glucose and fat in your blood, instead of in your cells. The blood has no use for it; meanwhile your cells are starved of their energy source and protein can't be used to repair organs or muscles. Through the years, this internal imbalance can damage nerves and blood vessels, which can ultimately result in heart disease, stroke, blindness, kidney disease, nerve problems, gum infections, and amputations. The goal of diabetes treatment is to get sugar into the cells where it can be used, and out of the bloodstream where it's just going to wreak havoc.

Type Casting

Diabetes comes in one of three forms: type 1, type 2, and gestational diabetes.

Gestational diabetes can develop in the late stages of a woman's pregnancy, as a result of pregnancy hormones that prevent insulin from doing its job. Gestational diabetes occurs most frequently among African-American, Latina, and American Indian women, and among women who are overweight or have a family history of diabetes. Although this form of diabetes usually goes away after the baby is born, a woman who has had gestational diabetes has a 20- to 50-percent chance of developing diabetes in the next five to 10 years. She's also more likely to develop type 2 diabetes later in life.

Type 1 diabetes is an autoimmune disease—your immune system mistakenly attacks and destroys the cells in the pancreas where insulin is made. It's not clear why this happens, but, when it does, your body isn't able to make enough of its own insulin to keep your blood-sugar levels normal. People with type 1 diabetes require daily insulin injections to live. Because of this, type 1 diabetes was previously called insulin-dependent diabetes mellitus. You'll also hear it referred to as juvenile onset diabetes—because it usually occurred among children and adolescents—but it may be diagnosed among people at any age.

About 1 out of every 10 people with diabetes has type 1. A few Black Americans with type 1 diabetes develop a form that doesn't appear to actually be an autoimmune response. In these cases, the body's ability to make its own insulin—and, thus, the need for medication—may fluctuate. This type is strongly hereditary.

Type 2 diabetes is the most prevalent type of diabetes; nine out of every 10 people diagnosed with the disease have this type. For every six white Americans who have it, 10 African-Americans do. Though research has established that a person's likelihood of getting diabetes is strongly based on genetics, the exact cause of type 2 diabetes is not understood, but we do understand how it works: if you have type 2, your body either doesn't make enough insulin, which is called insulin deficiency, or the cells in the muscles, liver, and fat do not use insulin properly, which is called insulin resistance. (See sidebar on page 18.)

Type 2 diabetes was previously called either "non-insulin dependent diabetes"—because it was usually managed with pills instead of injections—or "adult-onset diabetes" because it developed in adults only. However, many people with type 2 diabetes have to take insulin injections to effectively manage blood glucose levels, and it has now reached epidemic proportions among our youth. Though there are similarities between types 1 and 2, it's important to remember that just because you're taking insulin shots, your diagnosis is not changed to type 1 diabetes.

Type 2 diabetes most often occurs in people who:

▶ **Are older than age 40.** As you age, the pancreas may not work as well.

▶ **Are overweight or physically inactive.** When you're heavy your cells become more resistant to insulin.

▶ **Have a family history of diabetes.** Other members of your family having diabetes makes you a prime candidate.

▶ **Have a history of diabetes during pregnancy.** Pregnancy hormones make your cells more resistant to insulin. After the baby is delivered, the hormones and blood-sugar levels go back to normal. But mama has to be careful about eating well and getting exercise, or she'll increase the likelihood that she'll develop type 2 diabetes sooner.

▶ **Have given birth to a baby who weighed more than 9 pounds.** Women giving birth to large babies might have had gestational diabetes, which is a risk factor for diabetes.

▶ **Are African-American, Latino American, or American Indian.** Researchers think this may be caused by the "thrifty" genes that helped our ancestors survive by increasing fat storage during periods of famine. But today, with food readily available, the ability to store fat only results in obesity.

▶ **Have impaired glucose tolerance.** This means you have blood glucose levels above normal but lower than a person with diabetes.

▶ **Have high blood pressure or high blood fats.** These conditions are associated with insulin resistance.

What Is Insulin Resistance?

Let's make an insulin metaphor: Think of insulin as the key that unlocks the doors of the muscle or fat cells, so that glucose can enter and be used for energy. If your body doesn't make enough insulin, that's called insulin deficiency, which means nothing much is knocking at those cell doors.

In insulin resistance, however, insulin is being made, but the muscle, liver, and fat cells don't use it properly. It's as if the cell doors no longer recognize insulin and won't open to allow glucose in. Or think of the cell as being hard-of-hearing, so it can't hear the insulin that's banging on the door. As insulin continues to knock at the cell door, the amount of glucose in the blood increases, while the cells are starved of energy. The energy-deprived cell sends a signal to the brain that it needs energy. The brain, thinking lack of insulin is the problem, sends a signal to the pancreas to release more. The insulin rushes into the bloodstream, only to find the other insulin there, still knocking to be let in, and a backup of blood sugar with no place to go.

Eventually, the cell will hear all that insulin knocking and open the door, allowing glucose in. But meanwhile the pancreas has been working overtime. Eventually it gets "tired" and is no longer able to produce the additional insulin necessary to get glucose into the cell. When insulin levels fall—and not enough can be produced to replace it—blood-sugar levels start to rise again.

The liver can also be resistant to insulin. Think of the liver as a glucose storage tank. It helps control glucose levels in the blood between one meal and the next, preventing blood-sugar levels from going too high or too low. After you eat, glucose levels are high enough, so insulin prevents the liver from releasing more. But when it's been a while since you've had a meal and your blood sugar starts to drop, the liver releases more. However, when the liver is resistant to insulin, it will release stored glucose even when it's not needed, flooding the blood with sugar.

How Is Diabetes Diagnosed?

Diabetes is a fairly "invisible" disease, and the symptoms are sometimes subtle. It's easy to have one or two symptoms—feeling tired, contracting infections—and think nothing of them. But if you have one of the other risk factor, that makes you a prime candidate for diabetes—*and* you have some of the symptoms that follow, you should definitely have your blood sugar checked.

Symptoms of high blood glucose include:

 ⊳ Increased thirst

 ⊳ Extreme hunger

 ⊳ Frequent urination

 ⊳ Feeling tired

 ⊳ Itchy or dry skin

 ⊳ Slow-healing cuts or sores

 ⊳ More infections than usual

 ⊳ Tingling or numbness in hands or feet

 ⊳ Unexplained weight loss

 ⊳ Sudden vision changes

There are four different ways your doctor can determine if you have diabetes: A1C blood test, fasting blood glucose test, oral glucose tolerance test and casual blood glucose test. A person with diabetes will have measurements above normal on the A1C blood test, fasting blood glucose test and/or the oral glucose tolerance performed on two different days.

▸ **A1C blood tests** do not require fasting. The A1C test tells you what your average blood glucose level has been every day for the past 90 days. A person with diabetes will have an A1C measurement above 6.5 percent.

▸ **Fasting blood glucose tests** are done after an eight- to 12-hour period of going without food. A person without diabetes will have a fasting blood glucose measurement less than 100 milligrams/deciliter (mg/dL). A person with diabetes will have a fasting blood glucose measurement above 126 mg/dL. (People whose measurements fall between 100 and 126 are considered to have prediabetes.)

▸ **Oral glucose tolerance tests** measure your blood glucose up to five times in a three-hour period. First, a fasting blood glucose test is done. Then you drink a sweet liquid that contains 75 grams of glucose. Your blood glucose is then measured at 30 minutes, one hour, and two or three hours after the drink. A person with diabetes will have a two-hour measurement above 200 mg/dL.

▶ **Casual blood glucose tests** can be taken anytime during the day; it doesn't matter when you ate your last meal. If you have a casual measurement above 200 mg/dL plus symptoms of diabetes (extreme hunger, frequent urination and unexplained weight loss), you will likely be diagnosed with the disease.

─❦─

Prediabetes

If your blood glucose levels are higher than normal, but not high enough to be classified as diabetes, you have a condition called prediabetes. Just as the word implies, prediabetes exists before the actual onset of diabetes. But while prediabetes is definitely a risk factor for type 2, a number of research studies show that having prediabetes doesn't mean a diabetes diagnosis is inevitable.

. Take the Diabetes Prevention Program (DPP) study. It involved more than 3,000 people, half of whom were people of color—Black, American Indian, Asian, Pacific Islander, or Latino. All of them were overweight and had higher-than-normal blood glucose—prediabetes.

The DPP tested two approaches to preventing prediabetes from turning to type 2 diabetes: They had one group modify their lifestyle, lowering their intake of fat and calories and exercising about 30 minutes a day, five days a week. A second group used the diabetes drug metformin (commonly known as Glucophage). Those who took the drug received standard information on exercise and diet, but weren't required to modify their dietary or exercise habits. When the study ended, the people in the lifestyle modification group had lost an average of 15 pounds—reducing one of the main risk factors for diabetes. In fact, they reduced their risk of getting type 2 diabetes by 58 percent. People older than age 60 reduced their risk by 71 percent.

For many folks, a diagnosis of prediabetes can be worrisome. I like to think of it as an opportunity—your chance to prevent or delay the onset of diabetes. As the DPP study proves, diabetes isn't a given— even if you have prediabetes and other risk factors. It does mean that you have to take that prediabetes diagnosis seriously and actively work to prevent your blood-sugar levels from going any higher. If you are willing to change your lifestyle a little—lose a few pounds, fit in a workout—you can prevent diabetes.

─❦─

Myths, Mystery, and Misinformation

For all that we do know about how diabetes affects the body and how it can be prevented, some aspects of diabetes are still surrounded by a great deal of mythology and misinformation. Listening to old-wives' tales or Uncle Pookie's take on the best way to treat your condition can just confuse the issue even more. The more you know for sure, the better able you will be to successfully treat your condition. Here are some of the most common myths about diabetes—along with information you can rely on. Trust me.

Myth: If you eat too many sweets, you'll get diabetes.

Fact: Diabetes isn't caused by eating too much sugar; it's caused by genetics and lifestyle factors. However, eating foods high in sugar, fat, and calories can cause you to become overweight, which increases your risk of developing type 2 diabetes.

Myth: Type 1 diabetes is more serious than type 2 diabetes.

Fact: All types of diabetes are serious. Type 1 and type 2 involve elevated blood glucose levels which can lead to serious complications such as nerve damage, foot ulcers, amputation, kidney failure, heart disease, stroke, and blindness.

Myth: If you don't take diabetes medicine, your diabetes must not be serious.

Fact: Not everyone who has diabetes takes medicine for it. If your body produces some insulin, losing weight, adopting healthy eating, and getting regular physical activity can help insulin work more effectively. However, even if you don't take medicine now, you need to keep a close eye on your condition. Diabetes does change through time, and diabetes medicine may be needed later.

Myth: If you get diabetes, insulin will cure it.

Fact: Insulin doesn't cure diabetes. It helps to control diabetes by keeping the blood glucose from rising. At this point, there is no cure, only medicines and lifestyle changes that can help you manage it better.

Myth: If you have diabetes you can expect to lose your sight and limbs eventually.

Fact: Having diabetes doesn't mean you're doomed to sightlessness or amputations. Keeping your diabetes under control can prevent the most serious complications.

Myth: Dessert is off limits if you have diabetes.

Fact: While eating too many sugary foods is not a good idea, you can have an occasional dessert. It should be counted as part of your total carbohydrate intake for the day. Meaning, if you plan to have a piece of wedding cake, limit the bread, potatos, and other carbs you eat that day.

Myth: If you love bread, potatoes, and pasta, you're out of luck. Carbs and starches are off-limits if you have diabetes.

Fact: Carbohydrates and starches are part of a healthy diet—even for people with diabetes. You have to control your portions, but you can enjoy a nice pasta salad or a few potatoes if you like.

Myth: You can cure diabetes with the right diet.

Fact: A healthy diet and exercise can reduce your chances of getting diabetes, but once you have it, you have it. Diabetes is a lifelong disease that has no cure. However, with proper management (that includes that healthy diet again) it can be well controlled.

Frankly, diabetes can be a difficult disease to understand. You can't see it or feel it, but it's there, silently doing all kinds of things in your body. Then there are the different types of diabetes and, you'll soon discover, all the various treatment methods. Add to that all the myths and misinterpretations associated with the disease, and you have a formula for confusion.

But the fact that you're holding this book and have read this far means that you are serious about getting the best advice you can find to help you manage your disease. If you're just as dilligent about finding the best care providers and being proactive about following sound medical advice, you'll find that diabetes isn't so terribly confusing after all—and it's something you can manage quite effectively.

Power Points

☞ Diabetes happens when your body isn't using insulin properly. If you can get your blood sugar under control, you can control the disease. There is no cure for diabetes. Yet.

☞ Managing your diabetes carefully, you can avoid damage to your nerves and blood vessels—which can result in complications including heart disease, stroke, blindness, kidney disease, nerve problems, gum infections, and amputations.

☞ If you are diagnosed with prediabetes, you can prevent or delay type 2 diabetes by eating healthy meals and managing your weight.

☞ See your doctor right away if you notice symptoms of diabetes—extreme hunger, frequent urination, increased thirst, and unexplained weight loss. The sooner you're diagnosed the sooner you are able to start a diabetes management lifestyle.

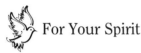 For Your Spirit

We Shall Overcome

Once upon a time, diabetes was a killer. People wasted away from a disease that no one understood and that nothing seemed to cure or prevent. In 1921, Frederick Banting and his assistant Charles Best figured out that a pancreatic extract called insulin could help. In 1940, the American Diabetes Association was founded to help educate people and raise money for research toward a cure. Through the years, doctors and researchers discovered new medicines to treat the disease; nutrition experts continued to search for the ideal diabetic diet. New ways to test blood sugar were invented. And research is ongoing. Progress is being made.

Once a devastating diagnosis that meant deprivation during life and a hastened death, diabetes is now neither a life sentence nor a death sentence, but a disease that can be overcome.

We know all about overcoming. As Black people in America, our "once upon a time" was far from a fairy tale. If you know even a little history, you know that our grandparents and theirs suffered in conditions that they didn't know how to remedy, that they could hardly imagine would change. But individuals had brave, bold ideas for change. Organizations were formed to support our efforts toward a better life. People fought for—and made—important gains. The work is ongoing, but progress is being made.

When we look at history—whether it's health history or social history—we see so many stories of survival. Just as diabetes is transferred in our genes, our ability to survive is just as strongly rooted genetically. And that knowledge can serve as our inspiration as we face the diagnosis of a disease that has no cure. When we remember our deeply rooted survival instincts—and tap into them—we can gain the inspiration we need to take action toward our own self care.

Action is key. Survival is not a passive thing. It takes strategy. (Figuring out how to revamp your holiday dinner to a more diabetes-friendly one.) It requires passion. (Dedicating yourself to doing your 30-minute workout every day.) It means tapping into your resources. (Joining a diabetes support group or reaching out to find the best endocrinologist you can find.) And it demands faith—faith that your efforts will be rewarded and that the strength you inherited from the people who came before you will prevail. Using all the skills and blessings that have been given to you, you will soon discover that, just like any other challenge you encounter, diabetes can be overcome.

2 YOUR DIABETES DREAM TEAM

Because diabetes is a disease that affects so many parts of your body (your eyes, your pancreas, your kidneys, your feet) and demands attention in so many aspects of your daily life (your diet, your fitness routine, your medication schedule), one single doctor—even a great one—may not be able to provide you with the level of detailed care you need. You will quickly see that having a group of people working *with* and *for* you can ease the burden of trying to make the best decisions for your own care.

Just as the "Dream Team" of the 1992 Olympics had their eyes on a gold medal, your diabetes dream team has a goal as well. Their mission is to help you stay as healthy as possible as you manage your diabetes. But like the basketball team, your team will need to learn to work well together. That's the job of the most important member of the team—the captain.

Every team has a captain who motivates the team to work together and makes sure everyone is on the same page. The captain of your dream team is you. That's right, *you.*

I can hear you protesting now: *I'm not a doctor. I don't know anything about diabetes. If I'm running the show, what am I paying all these medical people for?* No, you're not a doctor, but you are the only one who can describe how you feel. You are the one who tracks your blood-sugar levels and monitors the results, who takes your diabetes medications or insulin injections. You're the one who decides what you are going to eat and when you will exercise. No one can do all that but you—and "all that" is a crucial part of your care. All that must also be communicated among the various other members of your team so that they can do their jobs better. And because we're talking about your body, only you can take on that role.

As team captain, you are responsible for talking openly and honestly with your team members. You've got to be sure that the left hand knows what the right hand is doing. If you are working within a large, organized, and inter-connected healthcare system, chances are that your records are available to different members of your team. But you can't guarantee that your primary doctor has pulled up a test your diabetes specialist ordered, or vice versa. You're going to have to make sure that everyone is communicating appropriately. That means you've got to speak up.

There may be times when one doctor recommends one thing, and another care-provider says something else. Unless you actually are a health professional, it may be difficult for you to decide for yourself which way to turn. In that case, your task is to follow up, asking each of your caregivers to talk to you about the pros and cons of the recommendations they've made. You may need to get them to talk to each other and come to consensus. Ultimately, though, all care decisions end with you because you're the one who must execute them.

As the captain, you need to know the game—in this case that means you've got to know about diabetes. That doesn't mean you need to start applying to medical school, but it does mean that you should do your homework and learn as much as you can about your disease. You've made a good start: you're reading this book. But you should continue to stay as up-to-date as possible on the latest diabetes news and information. Checking Websites like diabetes.org or dLife.com, going to diabetes expos and keeping up with health news can help. That will enable you to ask good questions during your appointments, and it will let your dream team members know you're taking your own care seriously. If they see you're bringing your A-game, they're going to be that much more attentive to you.

Speaking of Team Members....

Who are the people who make up your dream team? There may be quite a few professionals that you interact with as you navigate the world of diabetes care. At times it may seem like you do nothing but make visits to one of these folks or another. But when making appointments and shelling out those co-pays starts to feel like they're adding up to a major inconvenience, think of it this way: you are fortunate to have a team of people who are dedicated to helping you be well. And when it comes to keeping you healthy, the more the merrier.

Primary Care Doctor

In addition to a captain, every team has a coach. The coach of your dream team is your family practice doctor or an internist—known in health insurance terms as your primary care physician. That name says it all. This person is your first line of defense—your go-to person when you have any kind of physical illness. He or she will examine you, assess your condition, order tests, and make recommendations for your care. The internist can diagnose diabetes or pre-diabetes, prescribe treatment, and suggest lifestyle and diet changes that will help you. She may have a great deal of experience caring for patients with diabetes and have developed an expertise in diabetes care. Or she may refer you to a specialist for diabetes-specific care. As your coach, your primary doctor may manage and coordinate information from other team members and help you make the decisions based on input from each of them.

See her for:

▶ An initial diagnosis of symptoms.

▶ Prescriptions for diabetes medications.

▶ Help in coordinating care among different practitioners.

▶ Referrals to specialists.

▶ Questions related to your general health.

▶ Advice for communicating with other specialists.

Endocrinologist

Endocrinologists specialize in hormonal illnesses and glandular problems—thyroid, pancreas, ovaries, adrenal glands, and everything in between. As gland experts, they're accustomed to dealing with the complex interactions among the different systems of the body. And because diabetes is basically a hormone imbalance related to the way your pancreas produces or processes insulin, diabetes is a specialty of many endocrinologists. Your primary doctor may refer you to an endocrinologist who can evaluate your condition if your diagnosis is complex—if you are on multiple medications, on an insulin pump, use more than one type of insulin, or just can't seem to get your condition under control. He can offer specialized recommendations for your medical treatment and monitor your condition carefully.

See him for:

▶ Diabetes specific questions.

▶ Diagnosis and treatment of diabetes complications.

▶ Prescriptions for diabetes medications and other treatments—and adjustments to those.

▶ A close, regular evaluation of changes in your condition, your blood-sugar levels, your other symptoms.

▶ Solutions to side effects of medications.

Nurse

They're often seen as peripheral figures, but registered nurses (RNs) are important members of your team and vital to your diabetes care. Diabetes nurse educators or diabetes nurse practitioners are RNs who have received special training in caring for and educating diabetes patients. Many of them can tell you almost as much about your illness as your doctor (though their advise is no substitute for a doctor's regular care), including how to take your medications, give yourself insulin, monitor your blood sugars, recognize symptoms of high and low blood sugars, and how to handle sick days.

See her for:

▶ Detailed questions that your primary doc may be too busy to answer.

▶ Questions that arise between office visits.

▶ Information about how and when to take your medication.

▶ Explanations of your doctor's orders.

Registered Dietitians (RDs)

The relationship between diabetes and what, when, and how you eat is critical. For that reason, your doctor may suggest that you visit a dietitian for help better managing your diabetes diet. A registered dietitian—a nutrition specialist who has passed a national exam, completed an internship and, in many cases, earned a master's degree in the field—is trained in the science of diet modifications to help patients reach optimal health and to control illnesses such as diabetes. An RD, especially one who has been trained as a Certified Diabetes Educator (CDE), can help you to understand how food affects your diabetes and how to make dietary modifications that increase your wellness.

See him for:

▶ Explanations of the food-guide pyramid, glycemic index, carb-content of foods.

▶ Information on the relationship between medication, activity, and diet.

▶ Information on making diabetes-friendly meals at home and plans for eating out.

▶ Assistance for developing a diabetes meal plan.

▶ Questions about food labels and basic nutrition principles.

▶ Assistance with weight-loss diets.

Podiatrist

Doctors of Podiatric Medicine (DPM)—or foot doctors, as most of us know them—see a disproportionate number of diabetes patients because of the impact diabetes can have on the feet. Diabetes affects the nerves and blood circulation, making your feet and lower legs vulnerable to injury or infection. For example, a small sore can become a serious infection because the disease decreases your ability to fight infection. The tiniest untended injury—say, you nip yourself while you're clipping your nails—can worsen until you wind up facing an amputation. In order to help you avoid that drama, a podiatrist will examine your feet and provide immediate treatment for any foot and lower-leg problems that you experience. But you must examine your feet every day, without fail, so that you can alert your podiatrist right away to any problems you notice.

See her for:

▶ Regular checks on your feet.

▶ Having your nails clipped or your calluses and corns attended to.

▶ Any signs that you're experiencing neuropathy—tingling in the limbs that indicates nerve damage.

▶ Questions about and recommendations for the healthiest shoes, socks, and foot care products.

Ophthalmologist

Diabetes affects the blood vessels of the eyes and can cause vision problems, and even blindness, if left unaddressed. As a person with diabetes, you've probably already been encouraged to see your eye doctor at least once a year. Go more frequently if you are experiencing vision problems or if your vision suddenly worsens. And don't confuse the ophthalmologist with an optometrist. The former is a physician who can diagnose and treat eye disease; the other is primarily a vision-correction specialist.

See him for:

▶ Regular eye exams and diagnoses.

▶ An annual dilated eye exam.

▶ Treatment of diabetes-related eye conditions.

Dentist

It's important for everyone to have their mouth, teeth, and gums checked regularly, but people with diabetes should be even more diligent about dental care because they're at a greater risk for oral problems such as gum disease (gingivitis and periodontal disease), tongue swelling, fungal infections, and chronic mouth sores. While the average person is encouraged to see a dentist at least twice a year, you should go more often if you have been diagnosed with gum disease. Look for a dentist with either DDS (Doctor of Dental Surgery) or DMD (Doctor of Dental Medicine) behind his name, and ask if he has experience treating diabetes patients.

See her for:

▶ Sores in and around the mouth.

▶ Careful, regular cleaning of the teeth and gums.

▶ Treatment of gum disease and infection.

Mental Health Specialists

Diabetes—or any chronic disease—can have a profound impact on your mental and emotional well-being. Coping with the daily challenges that come with the disease can make you feel defeated, depressed, angry or sad. If you've begun to have such feelings—especially if they're lingering or deepening—you may want to see someone who can help you make sense of your diagnosis and cope with the long-term effects. Depending on the nature of your concerns, you'll choose:

▶ A psychiatrist, a medical doctor who can prescribe medication, talk therapy, or other kinds of therapies to ease your mood and mindset.

▶ A psychologist, a talk therapist who can offer activities and suggestions to help you manage your feelings and moods.

▶ A social worker who will deal with the impact your disease has on your moods and your family. She can also help you find resources to support your care and help you manage the practical aspects of living with diabetes.

There are any number of approaches to psychology and psychiatry, so do some research before you go to find out if your chosen counselor's approach feels comfortable to you.

See him for:

▶ Assistance in coping with feelings of depression, hopelessness, uncontrolled anger, and resentment.

▶ Developing the disciplines and habits that will help you stick to your diabetes meal plan.

▶ Advice on how to speak to—or speak up to—doctors.

▶ Advice on dealing with any practical, social, or family problem related to your condition.

Pharmacist

You'll see *a lot* of this guy if you end up taking oral or injected medication. At least once a month, unless you have your meds delivered by mail, you'll visit a drug store to get your medicine. That's a great opportunity for you to ask questions about your medication options. Just because a pharmacist works in a place that also sells magazines, snacks, and nail polish doesn't mean he or she is not a professional. A pharmacist is trained and licensed to understand, prepare, and dispense medication.

See her for:

▶ Questions about side effects and drug interactions.

▶ Generic and alternate drug options.

Exercise Physiologist

These professionally certified health care specialists are trained to understand the way exercise affects the body and how exercise is performed. Because exercise is an important part of diabetes treatment—especially in helping control your blood-sugar levels and keeping your weight in check—you may be referred to an exercise physiologists who can develop a fitness program especially for you and teach you how to add activity to your daily regimen. Every fitness trainer is not an exercise physiologist, so be sure you ask about your trainer's credentials. A trainer who is certified by the American College of Sports Medicine (or the equivalent) probably has the qualifications for which you're looking.

See him for:

▶ Creating and sticking to a fitness plan.

▶ Advice on avoiding exercise injuries.

▶ One-on-one exercise coaching.

Diabetes Educators

All of the members of your dream team are professionals who are trained in their special areas of expertise—whether it's hormones, feet or teeth—and their professional education will have included basic information on the needs of diabetes patients. But if your nurse, dietitian, psychologist, or pharmacist is also a Certified Diabetes Educator, consider yourself especially fortunate. CDEs are healthcare pros—licensed in another field—who have sought rigorous training in educating people with diabetes. A diabetes educator will work with you to set health goals and come up with strategies for managing your condition well. When your dream team members are also diabetes educators—and if you're fortunate, several of the people on your team might—you can feel confident that your care advisors are truly knowledgeable in teaching diabetes self-management.

Managing Your Team

When you look back over the list of team members, you see a *lot* of different people, different specialties, and different approaches. It might be easier if these folks worked as a team in the same office, communicating and coordinating with each other about your care. Unfortunately, that won't always be the case. All your care providers may not even know each other. That means it's going to be your job as team captain to work with all these folks to make sure that the advice you're being given is coordinated.

You'll need to be sure to note what you're being told in one office, so you can relate that information to the other caregivers. For example, if your endocrinologist prescribes medication to be taken a certain way, your dietitian needs to know exactly how and when you're to take the medicine, so she'll know when your meals should be scheduled. Your exercise physiologist may need to know if you've been given special instructions by your podiatrist. And so on. You get the picture.

Occasionally, you may get conflicting opinions about treatment or other aspects of your diabetes self-care. It's frustrating to have one person tell you one thing and another tell you something else—and it may be tempting to flip a coin and pick one over the other, or to ignore both and take matters into your own hands. Resist that temptation. Instead, start asking questions. Your goal is not to pit one caregiver against another, but for you to understand not only what you're being told but why. What is the thinking behind the advice you're being given?

Let's make up a scenario. Say you're at your appointment with your dietitian and she's talking about meal schedules. You check your diabetes notebook for notes from visits with other doctors to see if any of them said anything about eating or diet. You might tell your RD: "My endocrinologist told me it doesn't matter when I eat as long as I take my insulin?

"Absolutely not true!" she says. "Your meal schedule can have a huge impact on how and when you take your insulin."

You temptation might be to stop right there and either take her advice and ignore the endocrinologist or decide the MD must know better and that you'll ignore the dietitian instead. A better approach is to keep asking questions.

How can what I eat affect the insulin? What does the timing of my meals have to do with it? Why do you think the doctor would say that? Does it depend on the specific type of insulin? Keep asking and asking until it makes sense to you. If you're still conflicted, make a note to call the endocrinologist's office and ask the same questions. There may be a point at which you need to ask the two practitioners to talk to each other, hash it out between themselves and get back to you with an answer. Just know that you're going to be the one to take the lead on that. And, even if you feel uncomfortable or inconvenienced by doing it, you must. It's your health after all. And you are the captain of your personal healthcare dream team.

You can probably already see how this is going to tap all your communication and organization skills. Don't worry that you're not going to be able to manage all the medical jargon or remember what one doctor or the other said. The most important thing you can do is to ask questions if you're uncertain about anything any of the doctors tell you. And keep asking until you really understand what you're being told. The better you grasp things, the easier it will be to relate that information to the next team member.

Here's a helpful hint: keep a diabetes notebook or journal and take it with you to every appointment. Use it to jot down notes and instructions that your care provider gives you. Then you can refer to it when you see your next doctor or care provider. Also use it to make note of questions you want to ask, changes in symptoms, or anything that arises between office visits. A dedicated journal will go a long way in helping you feel on top of the information you're being given. It's also a good place to keep track of your "team roster"—names, addresses, and phone numbers of all your care givers.

Power Points

🖘 Diabetes affects many parts of your body such as your eyes, kidneys, and feet—which is why you need a team of healthcare professionals.

🖘 Primary care doctors, endocrinologists, nurses, dietitians, ophthalmologists, podiatrists, and pharmacists can all be part of your diabetes dream team.

🖘 Certified Diabetes Educators are healthcare professionals who specialize in providing care and education to people with diabetes.

🖘 You are the captain of your team.

🖘 Communication is key when working with a team of caregivers.

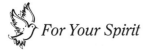 *For Your Spirit*

Put Your Hand in the Hand

It's pretty common knowledge that African-American people have a rather tenuous relationship with the healthcare system. And understandably so. Since our arrival in America, we've received the worst possible care. As slaves, if we saw a doctor, it may have been the same guy who took care of the cows and mules on the plantation. Then there was the notorious Tuskegee experiment, where poor African-American men were unknowingly used as guinea pigs—allowed to live with deadly syphilis infections so that doctors could see the progression of the disease. The segregated healthcare system in the Jim Crow era left many families with stories of loved ones who were refused treatment at white hospitals. And in more recent times, people in very urban and very rural communities have had to cope with the lack of qualified doctors, overcrowded clinics, the closing of hospitals in our neighborhoods and lack of access to specialized care. Add to that the complexities of the insurance system, which seems to stymie everyone, and you can see why we'd have a love-hate relationship with the healthcare system and remain a bit wary of doctors.

But if we pull away from the help that is available to us—if we don't learn to trust the people who are trying to provide us care, then we're condemning ourselves to a continued history of poor health. Our community can't afford that.

When it comes to care, if you're not a healthcare professional yourself, you have to put yourself in the hands of the experts. But that doesn't mean you do so blindly. It's a matter of having faith but also being wise.

The first step is to go within to see if you can figure out the origin of your discomfort or mistrust. Have you always disliked doctors' offices? Are you afraid of being diagnosed? Where did you pick up that fear? Are you haunted by stories of people who had bad experiences in the healthcare system? If your fears and discomfort are getting in the way of seeking care, you may want to talk with your mental health counselor, your spiritual advisor, or some other trusted person to help you face and overcome your fears.

Also, seek out care providers with whom you resonate. If you just don't like or trust your doctor, you're less likely to make appointments, less likely to follow his instructions, and less likely to feel comfortable asking questions or pursuing the information you need. It can be tricky to switch docs, depending on your healthcare plan, but if your spirit isn't connecting with the doctor you have, that's a signal that you may need to look into making a change. Ask friends and colleagues to recommend a good, well-qualified doctor.

Ultimately, seeking care is an act of faith and a commitment to trust the person offering you care. In order to put yourself in someone's hands, you may first have to say a prayer and do some meditation. Ask Spirit to send you to the people who can best help you take care of yourself. Be still and listen for the guidance that you can feel in your heart. Act on the best advice of the people who have been sent to you offering good help. And trust that, ultimately, your care is in good hands.

3 DITCHING "DENIABETES"

You've been tired lately. And your vision isn't what it used to be. You're always thirsty—which means you've been running to the bathroom a lot. But these are little things—not even worth mentioning to your doctor. So you are shocked when, at your annual checkup, your provider tells you your blood sugar is too high. "Unfortunately, it's diabetes," he tells you. "We need to decide on the best course of action."

What's your response?

1. "Diabetes? No, I'm not claiming that."
2. "Diabetes runs in my family, but I don't think I have it."
3. "So I've got a touch of sugar. No big deal."
4. "Sugar? That's probably just that cake my wife made on Sunday."

Any of these responses sound familiar? If so, you're not alone. A lot of people take the less-is-more, wait-and-see, or it-can't-be me approach to dealing with diabetes. And many of us exercise our faith by affirming that we "won't claim" something like diabetes—believing that if we pray hard enough and have enough faith, God will just make it go away.

The reality is that there is no such thing as a "touch of sugar." You either have diabetes or you don't—and wishing it away and praying it away is probably not going to make it actually *go* away. Four million—yes, *million*—African-Americans have been diagnosed with the disease and "not claiming it" hasn't cured a one of them.

Before you get alarmed, no one is saying you should lose your religion over diabetes. Should you have faith? Sure. Does positive thinking help? Absolutely. Must you pray? Daily—hourly if you like. And it will help. Research points to the benefits of prayer and a positive mental attitude for physical healing. But for too many of us, "not claiming it" is the extent of our self-care. We keep eating whatever we want, drinking whatever we want, avoiding our medications, and living our couch-potato lifestyle, hoping and praying that the disease will just disappear. But you know what they say about "faith without works...." That's not how you want to end up, is it?

The good news is that diabetes doesn't have to put you in the grave. Though there's no cure yet for diabetes, it is a very manageable disease. And if you're willing to eat well, get active, work with good health professionals—and, yes, keep the faith—you can live a rich, sweet life with diabetes. That's what this book is all about: accepting, with grace, the challenge of diabetes and using your faith and all your God-given resources to manage the disease. The pages that follow will show you how.

Double Diagnosis

If you've been told you have diabetes and you don't do anything about it right away, you may actually have two diseases: diabetes and "deniabetes." *Diabetes* symptoms include thirst, frequent urination, fatigue, and blurred vision. Symptoms of *deniabetes*—denial of diabetes—include a refusal to admit that you have the previously mentioned symptoms; an unwillingness to accept a diabetes diagnosis when your doctor hands it to you; and a lack of attention to the medical, dietary, exercise, and other recommendations your healthcare providers offer to help you treat and manage the disease.

Unfortunately, the two diseases don't cancel each other out. Denying you have diabetes won't make it go away. In fact, if you don't cure yourself of deniabetes, your diabetes is likely to get worse. If diabetes goes uncontrolled long enough, it can lead to all kinds of complications that can have devastating effects on your eyes, kidneys, limbs, and heart. The good news is that deniabetes is absolutely curable and diabetes itself is not a death sentence. Once your deniabetes is managed, you can begin to manage your diabetes much more effectively.

Stages of Denial

Denial comes in different guises. The first is **simple denial**. Simple denial is strong and clear: you completely refuse to believe that something has happened. It's often this basic form of denial that prompts people to ask for additional tests or a second opinion—which is never a bad idea. But when the diagnosis is undeniable, you may do yourself a disservice when you "just say no" and leave it at that. I often hear the phrase "I'm not claiming it" from people who are confronted with an unwelcome diagnosis or other life challenge. I understand that they're using it as an affirmation of faith. But there's a difference between refusing to let a situation bring you down and completely ignoring it altogether. The latter can be deadly.

There are also folks who understand that they are sick but deny the seriousness of their condition. Mentally reducing the consequences of the diagnosis is known as **minimization**. This type of denial may happen if you know you have diabetes but tell yourself "it isn't that bad." This perspective can also be a result of a doctor trying to break the news to you gently. If she says your "blood sugar is a touch high," you may take that to mean you have a mild form of diabetes—one that doesn't need much attention from you. You may minimize your condition if you don't have enough information to fully grasp the seriousness of the disease.

Another form of denial is known as **transference**. That's when you know you have diabetes and you recognize that it's something to take seriously, but feel that "taking it seriously" is someone else's job. It's denying that you are responsible for taking care of yourself. If you're "transferring," you may turn to your spouse, grown child, or someone else close to you to order your prescriptions, prepare appropriate meals, or otherwise manage your condition.

You might be in denial if you hear yourself saying or thinking:

> *"One bite of pie won't hurt."*
> *"This sore will heal by itself."*
> *"At least I only take pills, not shots."*
> *"I'll go to the doctor later."*
> *"I only have borderline diabetes."*
> *"I'm to busy to do it."*
> *"My diabetes isn't serious."*
> *"My insurance doesn't cover that."*
> *"My blood sugar is just a little high."*
> *"Everybody has to die from something."*

Psychologically, denial isn't necessarily a bad thing. Your brain uses denial as a defense mechanism to keep you emotionally safe; it prevents you from feeling anxiety when you're stressed. As a temporary mental state, denial helps protect you from thoughts that are painful or uncomfortable, and it keeps you from feeling totally dejected and depressed when you receive unfortunate news. It can buy you time to accept your situation and figure out a way to take self-protective action. The trouble comes in when it moves beyond a *temporary* state. If you dwell in a state of denial about a chronic condition—one that needs your regular attention and decisive action—it can interfere with your ability to live well and survive. The longer it takes you to move from the healthy, normal denial phase into acceptance and action, the more you put your long-term health at risk.

The first step in accepting diabetes is accepting the fact that denial may just be a natural part of the process. We all experience denial at some point in our lives and, frankly, just about everybody experiences a little denial after a diabetes diagnosis. For even the most self-aware, health-conscious person, acceptance of a chronic condition is rarely instantaneous. It is a pretty big deal. After all, you are accepting a major loss—the loss of your "normal" life. If you think of it that way—as a cause for grief—it's easy to see why denial would be a natural response to your diagnosis. But getting through any form of grief is a process. If you remember the stages of the grieving process, you'll note that denial is usually the first stage, followed by anger, bargaining, depression and, finally, acceptance. Grief experts warn that you can expect to cycle in and out of the stages of grief—including denial—several times on your path to acceptance.

Breaking Free

When you are learning to cope with diabetes, you may encounter triggers that back-track. When you feel fine, your blood sugar is under control, and you aren't experiencing any symptoms, it can be easy to forget all about your diabetes. Holidays, family gatherings, or even the act of grocery shopping can cause you to fall back into your former habits—having that second slice of pecan pie or dropping a quart of butter pecan ice cream into your grocery cart. Denial often happens because, by nature, humans are afraid of any change. Just the thought of having to alter your lifestyle can cause you to panic—*I'll have to empty my sugar jar into the garbage! I'll have to get up in the middle of the night to go exercise!* Your self-protection mechanism kicks in to ease your fear and—oops—there you are, right back in denial.

You can break free from denial by taking these steps:

▶ **Surround yourself with truth tellers.** Find family members, doctors, diabetes-care advisors, or others in your community who are willing to work with you to keep you on track. Ask a member of your diabetes team about things you can do to take care of your diabetes. Ask a diabetes educator to help you develop a health plan. Find a fitness buddy who will exercise with you every day—and won't tempt you to go grab a muffin and a latte afterward. Look for and rely on your true friends—the ones who want you to do everything you can to stay healthy today and for many years to come.

▸ **Post your diabetes care plan and your health goals.** Work with your family, diabetes educator, or other supporters to develop a complete life plan that incorporates your diabetes care. Then post the highlights on the fridge, on the bathroom mirror, or beside your bed—anywhere you will see them and be reminded to stay on track.

▸ **Understand how diabetes works.** If you understand exactly how certain foods affect your blood sugar, then you're more likely to stop and think before you make your dessert selection. Having a clearer picture of how uncontrolled diabetes can affect your heart health, your kidney function, your ability to heal from a wound, can increase your sense of urgency when it comes to taking care of your health.

▸ **Keep an eye out for signs that denial is creeping up again.** Studies suggest that even when you have accurate information, a good support system and the best intentions in the world, you can still experience symptoms of denial. You have to watch for it all the time—and shoo it away every time it comes sneaking up.

It may take a while for you to fully release yourself from denial. And that's okay. Forgive yourself when you slip into it and keep moving on. One day at a time. That's the way to get through this.

Why me?

Even if you aren't in denial about diabetes, you may have other emotions, mental blocks, and hang-ups about the disease—that can get in the way of taking action toward your diabetes self-care. It's quite common to feel angry, guilty, sad, depressed, afraid, or anxious after a diabetes diagnosis. The goal is to acknowledge and accept your feelings. There is no right or wrong way to feel. If you're mad, you're mad. As long as you aren't taking it out on other people—or yourself—your anger is just a feeling. You also have to understand how your emotions can affect your self-care decisions. If you're too depressed to cook, you're less likely to eat diabetes-healthy food. If you can't get motivated to get out of bed, you're going to miss the benefits of exercising. So you have to get out of denial about your emotions as well as about your disease—and develop strategies for dealing with them in a positive way. Understanding your emotions will help you to work through them and live a healthy life with diabetes.

It may mean that you have to have a long talk with your doctor. She may be able to refer you to a counselor who can give you strategies for coping with your emotions. Counselors can give you techniques for changing your mindset, seeing your situation more objectively, and finding the motivation to take positive action toward your own care. Pastoral counselors may help you with this, as well. A spiritual approach may include praying for understanding and motivation as well as developing strategies for taking care of your "temple."

You have to learn to turn off the negative thinking as well. If, every day you tell yourself the worst is going to happen, you won't see anything but...the worst. Begin to take note of that little voice in your ear and be sure it's not filling your head with thoughts like the following:

▶ **What did I do to deserve this?** Some people believe health problems happen to those who deserve them. They think that if you receive a disease diagnosis, it must be a punishment for some moral defect. For those folks, accepting the idea that they have diabetes means that they have to accept that they have a character flaw so great that they deserve a disease. And who wants to think they're so terrible that God would select them for an affliction? But if that's your way of thinking—you deserve a disease—what's your motivation to work on managing the disease? You're either going to work yourself into a frenzy trying to fix the spiritual failing—and ignore the physical symptoms. Or you're going to give up: "God gave me diabetes. Nothing I can do this side of judgment day."

Diabetes results from something going awry in our bodies—not in our character or spirit. And the all-powerful God is also a loving and forgiving spirit in our lives. I like to think of God as the Spirit of helpfulness—sending resources, information and helpmates so that I can do everything possible on earth to take good care of myself. If you take this approach, you can constantly tell yourself, "This disease is not a punishment; it's a condition of life. And it's not my fault, but it's my responsibility to take care of it."

▶ **This is the worst thing that could ever happen to me.** Do you have memories of family members who went blind, suffered amputations, or ended up on dialysis because of diabetes? Or did your doctor make diabetes sound like a death sentence (as many did only a couple of decades ago)? If tragic family experiences or a no-hope doctor's words are your only frame of reference to diabetes, diabetes will seem like a disease to dread.

The cure for this fear is information. And the fact that you're reading this book says you're on the right path toward getting the information you need. There's more in the pages that follow. For now just know that diabetes research has resulted in new information and new treatments over the years. Today you have access to better technology, better glucose monitors, more convenient meal-planning methods. There's even the hope of an artificial pancreas that could eliminate the need for medications. These days, people understand that diabetes is quite manageable. You can live a long, healthy, happy, active life with the disease. Diabetes is far from the worst thing that can happen to you.

▶ **The doctor didn't make a big deal of it. Why should I?** If your doctor minimizes the seriousness of your illness, it can cause you to feel that it's not a big enough concern for you to attend to. Besides, you have enough on your plate as it is, right? If this is something that can go on the back burner, why shouldn't you leave it there? Well, because if you back-burner diabetes, it can simmer there until it boils over into a full-fledged crisis.

I'm not saying don't listen to your doctor. In fact, I'm saying listen very, very carefully. And the minute you hear the word diabetes or even pre-diabetes, start asking questions. *Lots* of questions. And look for ways to begin to manage your condition right away.

▶ **I just can't deal with it.** You've been good. You check your blood sugars, watch what you eat, take your medicine, and get your daily exercise. Every. Single. Day. And you're just about sick of it. Burnout happens when you start to feel frustrated as a result of continuously having to do the things you have to do to take care of yourself. Until it becomes a natural part of your daily lifestyle, your diabetes self care may seem like a series of new chores you have to do. And when you're burned out, you just don't have the motivation you need to take care of yourself.

When you start to feel burned out tell yourself this truth: *I don't have to do any of this any more.* Because you don't. You can toss your glucose monitor and insulin in the garbage, grab the remote and a box of Twinkies and watch re-runs all day long. You can. But then ask yourself this question: *If I stop managing my diabetes, what will happen?* Consider the damage to your health. Think about the complications that can arise. Think about what your increasing illness will mean for the people you love. Then ask yourself: *Is it worth it to quit?*

Let me answer that last one for you: *No.* It's not worth it to quit because your life is priceless. You were put on this earth with a purpose and you are destined to live out your days accomplishing your mission and enjoying the good fruits of your work. You want all the time you can get to enjoy the life Creator has given you—and the good health that goes along with it.

Signs, Symptoms, and Solutions

	Reasons	Signs	Solutions
Depression	You can't cure it. You're facing a lifelong chronic condition. You tried to avoid diabetes and failed. You believe you must give up your favorite foods and way of life. You're afraid that diabetes threatened your health and lifespan. You feel you have no control over the complications of diabetes. You can't afford diabetes medication or the health care.	You feel sad or empty every day. You feel guilty or worthless. You don't look forward to anything; don't get pleasure from anything. Have trouble concentrating. Have trouble sleeping or sleep too much. Feel sluggish and tired everyday. Weight and appetite changes—poor appetite and weight loss or increased appetite and weight gain. You think about death and dying everyday.	Take it seriously. Studies show that people with diabetes have more depression than the general public. Seek counseling. Your doctor can refer you to a mental health professional. Your clergy or spiritual advisor can refer you to a Christian mental health provider if you prefer. Accept treatment. There are many treatments and techniques available to help manage depression. Get a physical. Sometimes depression can be caused by physical aliments.
Fear	You know diabetes has complications such as blindness or amputation. You don't like shots. You know someone who died from diabetes or was on dialysis. You can't afford diabetes medication or health care.	Worry all the time about your blood glucose being too high or too low. You check it two or three times before or after a meal. Feel paralyzed and unable to take action. Feel obsessive about when and how much you eat the amount of food you eat and the time you eat. Feel there are foods that you must never eat. Avoid eating away from home.	Focus on the quality of your life as well as your blood glucose control. Get informed. The more you know, the less likely you are to feel afraid. Make plans. You'll feel more in control if you find ways to anticipate what you'll need. Use fear to motivate you to learn all you can about diabetes. Aim for progress not perfection. No one is perfect!

Signs, Symptoms, and Solutions (continued)

	Reasons	Signs	Solutions
Anxiety	You're not sure you're going to be able to manage taking care of your disease. You're afraid of all the medications you'll have to take. The diabetes diet means learning to cook a whole new way. You're not sure you're up to it.	Are irritable or jittery. Have difficulty concentrating. Get tired very easily. Have racing thoughts or your mind goes blank. Experience muscle tension. Have difficulty falling to sleep or staying asleep. Everything seems to worry you.	Use the techniques for dealing with depression (above). Talk to a mental health counselor. He may be able to give you tips specific to anxiety.

Power Points

☞ There is no such thing as a little sugar or a touch of sugar. Diabetes is diabetes.

☞ Continued denial keeps you from learning how to be healthy with diabetes.

☞ Education is the best defense against denial.

☞ After learning you have diabetes, you may feel shock, denial, anger, guilt, sadness, depression, fear, or anxiety.

☞ Acknowledge your denial or anxious feelings and learn how to deal with them in a positive way.

☞ Get help from a counselor if you feel overwhelmed by your emotions.

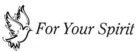 *For Your Spirit*

Truth Will Set You Free

"Truth is a divine thing, a friend more excellent than any human friend."

—St. Thomas Aquinas

We brace ourselves when the doctor comes in with our test results. We don't want to hear bad news. If we're given a clean bill of health, we're elated. But if hard news comes, we have actually been given a gift of another kind—the gift of a new beginning.

If you've been walking around with undiagnosed symptoms and a nagging sense that something is wrong, the truth of the doctor's diagnosis sets you free of that particular worry. You don't have to wonder any more. You know. And knowing frees you to start looking for ways to address the health issue you are facing.

Some theologians believe that truth is so pure and so divine that humans—sinners that we are—aren't capable of knowing the truth. Others believe we might come close to truth, but only through the divine intervention of God. St. Thomas Acquinas, the 13th-century theologian and philosopher, believed that humans have the God-given capacity to understand truth—and that we have an appetite for it. Deep in our souls, we want to know what is True.

Our souls may wonder, but sometimes our minds seem to want to ignore the inconvenient facts. When we are facing a challenge that looks like it might overwhelm us, it can seem simpler to just try to ignore it. *Maybe, if I don't look at it, it will go away.* Sometimes we don't want to delve in the dark places where truth resides—for fear that something frightening will reach out and bite us. And then too, if we are to accept a hard truth, we might have to do something about it. And most of us already have so much on our plates that it would seem nearly crazy to take on another job.

But scripture promises us that truth will not be a burden, but a lifesaver. In John 8:32–33, Jesus says, "If you continue in My word, then you are truly disciples of Mine; and you shall know the truth, and the truth will make you free."

When you know and accept your truth—you have diabetes—you can begin immediately to take steps to take care of yourself.

4 CHANGE YOUR MIND; CHANGE YOUR BEHAVIOR

While some people suffer from "deniabetes," others approach their diagnosis in just the opposite way—jumping right in to "fix it" quick. If you're one of these "Action Jacksons," it's admirable that you're willing to do whatever you can to help your health. That enthusiasm is great—as long as you can keep it up. The problem is that sometimes, through time, enthusiasm wanes and efforts falter. Eagerness and willingness are not quite all you need to build a healthy lifestyle that's consistent for a lifetime. Living healthy with diabetes requires as much mental and spiritual preparation as it does practical effort and willingness.

State of Mind

Every conscious action is the result of a forethought. You decide to do something, then you do it. Even a very spontaneous action involves at least a split-second of thought. The more serious your action, the more deeply you need to contemplate it. If you are thinking of making a change in your lifestyle—something permanent or nearly so—you have to think about it deeply enough and plan for it carefully enough to be able to sustain that change for an extended period of time.

Think of it this way: Deciding to go for a walk might be a spontaneous decision. You get the notion to take a stroll, you lace up your shoes and you're gone. You come back 30 minutes later, done. But if you decide that you are going to launch a new exercise routine that involves walking six days a week for 30 minutes, you have to consider how that's going to fit into your schedule, what you'll do if the weather is bad, what happens if you have a conflict or if you aren't feeling well. You may have to think about getting proper walking shoes or other workout clothes. You may have to plan your route; you'll want to take safety precautions. This is a much bigger commitment than walking around the block after dinner. And it takes more mental planning. You have to be in the right frame of mind—and the right place in your spirit—to approach lifestyle changes effectively. If you're not, the first thing that gets in your way may be the thing that stops you altogether.

That means that even if denial is the last thing on your mind—you're all ready to get to work on taking care of your diabetes—you still need to make some adjustments to your thinking.

Intention of Spirit

Beyond frame of mind, you must have the right *intention of spirit* to care for yourself properly, consistently, and wisely. What's the difference? You can tell yourself you're going to do something, and mentally *will* yourself to do it. But if your heart isn't really in it, your mind isn't likely to be able to rule. What's in your soul is the thing that is really going to move you and change you. So an intention that rises from your spirit adds strength to anything you mentally decide to do. Many of us know intellectually that we need to eat more green vegetables. We can remember and recite all the reasons why that's important. But if you don't *feel* like eating your broccoli, you're going to find a way not to do it. It's not until you really know in your soul that it's vital—and feel the calling from your soul to commit to it—that you are likely to stick with the commitment. If you are not in the right mental and spiritual place, nothing is going to happen.

Many faiths recommend spiritual strengthening through periods of prayer and fasting—sometimes a day, sometimes seven, sometimes more. (It's a spiritual practice that has to be modified for people with diabetes.) But if you've ever done it, you know it's more than just skipping a few meals. It's something you have to be mentally and spiritually prepared for, or you won't do it with a lot of success or without a lot of suffering. That's why the call is usually not just for fasting alone, but for "prayer and fasting"—because you need the prayer to move you through the fast successfully.

It's the same with any major endeavor: you need to be mentally and spiritually in tune in order to see it through with success. Nowhere is that more accurate than when you're trying to change your lifestyle to a healthier one.

Stages of Change

So what frame of mind do you need to be in to make a change? Well, psychologists who study how people experience change have come up with a theory that a true mental shift isn't actually one state of mind, but many.

The "Stages of Change" concept indicates that change isn't an "event." It's a process that takes several steps. Although sometimes it may seem like you just decided to change and it happened, just like that, if you backtrack and give it some *serious* thought you will discover that there was a process of making a decision to do the thing in the first place, then gearing yourself up, possibly adjusting your decision a little, then digging in to see how it works out.

For example, you don't just up and quit smoking one day—*bam.* Even if you go cold turkey, you've thought about it, you decided to do it, you picked a date, you got rid of your cigs, maybe you found a support group or looked for tips on how to quell your nicotine craving, perhaps you got some nicotine gum...and *then* you quit. And even after you quit, there's another process: You don't smoke one day. Then you don't smoke the next day. And you keep *not* smoking until you can safely say you've really quit. After all that you can say you've changed from a smoker to a nonsmoker.

A diabetes diagnosis necessarily requires lifestyle changes of some sort. Understanding how to get through the process of making those changes requires that you understand the unique thoughts and feelings that are going on at each stage in that process.

Pre-contemplation

The first stage in the Stages of Change concept is pre-contemplation. It's the "not even thinking about it" stage that comes before you have any idea that you need to change. If you're in the earliest phase of pre-contemplation, you won't even know it. For instance, someone might say, "Why should I change my diet? I only have a little sugar." Another word for this stage is denial. Maybe it is not denial of the problem but a denial of your responsibility for addressing the problem. When you hear a person say, "I know I'm heavy, but my whole family is heavy. Nothing I can do about it; it's in my genes," you know they're not ready to think about addressing their weight. They're in pre-contemplation.

But this is also the stage where you're beginning to get the information you need that will help open your eyes to the fact that maybe you need to look more deeply into your life and health. This is the *consciousness raising* part of the process. You're finding and learning new facts about your health condition. Reading a book like this one or talking to your doctor can be part of gaining greater awareness of changes you need to make in your lifestyle. Keeping a food journal or exercise log makes it absolutely clear how much you eat or how much (or how little) activity you get each day. Seeing your diet and exercise habits in black and white really makes you more aware of where you need to make adjustments.

If you are in the pre-contemplation stage, you may experience the following:

▸ **Taking stock.** You take a look at how your behavior affects the people around you and your environment in general. For example, you might consider how your poor glucose control worries your family, or inhibits your ability to drive safely or live alone.

▸ **Leaking emotions.** Maybe hearing you have diabetes makes you feel hopeless: "My dad had it and ended up on dialysis. It'll probably be the same for me." You may feel afraid, as many people do when they hear they have an incurable disease. Or you may just want to bury your head in the sand rather than face the hard work involved with managing diabetes. Sometimes before you can begin to address your condition, you need to address your underlying emotions first.

Contemplation

The next stage is contemplation. You know you have a health concern. Now you also know that you need to do something about it. But you haven't quite yet made the commitment to change. Though folks will say, "Well, why don't you just get up and get to it?"—it's not that simple, emotionally or spiritually. Even though it may be abundantly clear that you've got to make some moves, many things may stand in the way of making the *commitment* to do what you need to do. For instance, the thought of making a change may be overwhelming when you look at the energy, effort, or cost involved. Say you're planning to launch a weight-loss effort. That means adjusting your usual grocery list, changing your familiar recipes, shifting your schedule so you have time to cook instead of grabbing take-out—plus figuring out how to avoid the box of donuts at the office or Uncle Andrew's rich eggnog at Christmas. And you also need to look into the emotional reasons you may eat—stress, loneliness, the need for comfort. That's a lot of work. And if you've tried to make changes before and not been successful, you may feel discouraged about trying again—another emotion to overcome.

Contemplation is the stage in which you're gearing up for change—asking yourself if you are mentally, physically and emotionally ready. Having moved past pre-contemplation, you're telling yourself, "I need to do something about this weight" or "I've got to do a better job of monitoring my glucose"—but you haven't actually *done* anything about it. Some people "contemplate" for a few weeks; others may stay in this phase for years with no sense of urgency. And until you move out of contemplation stage, that's as far as it goes. You know you need to change but maybe you're scared to start or too overwhelmed to know where to begin. Regardless of the reason, the result is the same: you're sitting there, watching and waiting, while feelings of guilt, desperation, shame, and hopelessness develop. And, by the way, your health isn't improving, either.

In this stage, you've moved to a state of consciousness about your condition. You know you need to make lifestyle changes, but you're still working on fully embracing that fact and figuring out just what to do about it. Your thought process might include:

▶ **Re-evaluation.** You're coming to terms with the fact that changing means altering the way you see yourself and your life—changing your identity, so to speak. In this stage, you'll begin to picture your life *after* you've met your goal. For example, you begin to envision a daily routine that includes checking your blood sugar after meals and working out to keep yourself in good physical shape.

▶ **Looking back.** You may find yourself thinking about all the reasons you *don't* want to change. This may seem like backpedaling, but it's part of the process. At least now you're *thinking* about change. Before, it wasn't even on your mind.

▶ **Mourning.** You also have to deal with the "loss" of your lifestyle. Change means you have to let something go to make room for something new. But even if you are looking forward to your new healthy life, you may feel sad about the life you are moving away from.

Preparation

You've gone over it in your mind and you're clear: you've got to get a handle on your diabetes. Now all you've got to do is actively get ready to make the lifestyle changes required. That's when it's time for preparation. This is when you might start gathering tools to help you make the change, such as buying a glucose monitor so that when you start checking your blood sugars you have the tool you need, or getting cushioned socks and comfortable workout shoes. You're gathering all your resources—girding your loins, so to speak—so that you have everything you need to embark on your journey.

If you skip this stage, you're setting yourself up for failure, because you won't have the right tools for the job. If you've ever made a spur-of-the-moment New Years' resolution, you know what I mean. Without mental, spiritual, and practical preparation, your resolution is likely to falter before February. You can't make a change—and make it stick—until you're really, really ready. Preparation is the key.

▶ **Putting your toe in.** You can start to experiment with some of the changes you're going to make. For example, sampling some low-carb or low-sugar foods or experimenting with diabetes-friendly recipes might be a first step. You haven't launched your new meal plan completely, but you're getting a "taste" of what it will be like.

▶ **Gathering support.** If you've fully contemplated your lifestyle change, you may have come to the conclusion that it won't be easy to go it alone. Having a support system in place can really help. You may tell people around you that you are going to change your eating habits and lose weight, so that they can encourage you (or police you!). Or you may sign up with a walking group to make exercise easier and more enjoyable.

▶ **Planning, planning, planning.** What will you do when your best friend invites you to her annual dessert party? How will you get your exercise in during the frozen, snowy months? How will you manage your medications when you go on vacation? You're resourceful. You can figure out a solution for all these circumstances and more. But it helps when you've thought about it before you're faced with it. When you consider the good, the bad, and the inconvenient aspects of change, you're better able to prepare for whatever comes.

Action

The fourth stage of the change process is the one you've been waiting for: actually making the change. Though this step is easier if you've done the contemplation and preparation, it's still a challenging stage because this is where the real work begins. The action stage is when you actually begin to change your behaviors and habits.

For example, this is the stage where you put your exercise plan into effect. You contemplated what type of exercise would work for you; you prepared by investing in a "Y" membership. Now you take action by actually going to work out every day. Or let's say you've evaluated the changes you need to make in your diet and prepared by buying diabetes-friendly cookbooks. You're ready to act by cooking meals that are healthier options for your condition.

If you've spent enough time and energy on contemplation and preparation, the action stage may seem like the easiest one. You know what you need to do and you know why you need to do it. With long-lasting health as your motivation, you are ready and able to get started. And ultimately, getting started is simple: just do it.

▶ **The first step.** What will it be like to walk into that first exercise class? How is the low-carb dinner going to go over with your family? Will Aunt Betty's feelings be hurt if you pass on her pecan pie? Are *you* going to be able to pass on that pie? Changing your lifestyle means putting yourself in new environments and having new experiences— and facing new situations can make you a little nervous. The key is to take the first step. It's a leap of faith, but faith will carry you through.

▶ **Little by little.** If you decide that next Monday, you're going to start your medication, launch your exercise routine, and restock your pantry, you're likely to get overwhelmed. You're one person and that's a lot of life change to take on. You don't have to take action on everything at once. It's easier if you start one thing—say, your fitness plan—and get settled into that routine, before you start revamping your diet. Or you may decide to do a little bit now and build up to your ultimate goal. There's nothing wrong with taking a brisk walk three days a week until you build up your stamina and commitment to do it every day.

▶ **Call in the reinforcements.** When you're "good"—you stick to your plans—reward yourself as a way of reinforcing positive behavior. A treat doesn't need to be costly and it should never involve food. For instance, when you lose weight, you might buy a new pair of pants instead of celebrating with dessert.

▶ **Lead yourself not into temptation.** If you know you have a weakness for cookies, leave them in the store. Or, if your kids can't survive in a house without sweet treats, buy a sugar-free version for yourself. Do whatever you can to change your environment to promote your health goals and avoid being tempted to make undesirable choices.

Maintenance

Starting a health-improvement plan is challenging enough, but even more challenging is the fact that you have to *keep it up*. After your diabetes diagnosis, you'll be counting carbs (daily), exercising (daily), examining your feet (daily), and checking your blood sugars (several times a day). This is what the maintenance stage looks like. Change has become part of your daily routine. But it takes real energy to keep this up week after week.

Some folks believe that this stage is when you turn on the willpower—the sheer strength of will to carry out a course of action. But lasting life-style change doesn't depend on your will alone. Think of it this way: When you lift a heavy box, you can only hold it for so long. You may *want* or even *need* to hold it up, but eventually your strength will fail and the box will fall. Small spurts of willpower can help you (like when you will yourself to lace up your sneakers and go out for a walk) but if you depend on will-power alone for too long you will "drop the box."

Maintaining your healthy lifestyle requires you to make use of all the tools you gathered in the previous stages—motivation, faith, determination—in order to keep you moving forward. It requires you to work hard, constantly reevaluating your progress and making adjustments to meet any new challenges that come your way. This stage can last a short time or a lifetime.

▶ **Eyes on the prize.** Because diabetes can be an invisible disease—you're not breaking out, swelling up, or hurting anywhere—it's easy to minimize the need for constant care. Don't let yourself forget how important your new lifestyle is to your long-term health.

▶ **The new normal.** Eventually your new lifestyle changes won't be new; this will just be your lifestyle. You'll be able to talk about change in the past tense. The sooner you accept that this is just your life now—the more grace and good humor you can bring to your life with diabetes.

▶ **Seek support.** We don't go through life—or life changes—alone. At least we shouldn't. Now is the time to reach out to the folks who care about your wellness enough to encourage you to do the right thing. That may also mean putting a little space between yourself and friends or family members who don't fully support your efforts. This is no time for naysayers—no matter who they are. You may also consider joining a diabetes support group. It's a great way to meet people who share your concerns and experiences.

▶ **Fear of falling.** You're going to fall off the wagon. Everyone does at some point. But if you don't beat yourself up about it, you can come back with more knowledge and tools to stay in the maintenance stage. For example, if you spent all day at your cousin's wedding and didn't check your sugars or count your carbs, you'll realize that you should have planned better. And next time you will. General Colin Powell has said, "There are no secrets to success. It is the result of preparation, hard work, and learning from failure."

Some researchers believe that there is another stage, called ***termination***. However, when it comes to diabetes, the process of maintaining your health doesn't end—unless you're planning for a permanent "termination." (And we can't have that!) In most cases, you must not only keep up your routine, you have to stay in regular communication with your doctor and other health caregivers to be sure your diabetes is maintained properly.

As you travel through the stages of change you may not travel in a straight path. You may move from action back to contemplation; you may have to do some additional preparation in order to maintain your changes. You can skip stages or jump back several stages—a process called ***recycling***. You can expect to recycle through the stages several times before you make a permanent change.

Human Nature

All of this change stuff sounds pretty logical and fairly simple, doesn't it? And it certainly is—in theory. The reality is that it can be very difficult for us to make changes—even changes we want and need to make. We're creatures of habit; it's easiest to do the thing we've always done. So if you normally hit the snooze button three times before you roll out of bed, it'll be hard to put your feet on the floor at the first buzz of the alarm. You may manage to do it for a few days, but you will probably find yourself lapsing into your old habits—at least until the new habit becomes old hat.

It also comforts *other* people for you to stick to your routine. People like knowing what to expect; it can throw them off when you do something that seems out of character or counter to what's customary. So, if you always bake sweet potato pies for the family to munch on during Thanksgiving weekend, folks may balk if you switch to a healthier dessert. As much as folks may love you and support your effort—in theory—it can be hard for them to cope with the actual change you've made. They're not bad people. It's just human nature.

That's why it's important to move carefully and methodically into any lifestyle changes you need to make—even if you need to move fairly quickly to bring your diabetes under control. Following a process—one that begins with careful thought, planning and right intention—can help you move forward into a healthier lifestyle that lasts a long, healthy lifetime.

Power Points

☞ Change doesn't just start with action—you have to set your mind to it and reinforce it with a spiritual intention.

☞ Behavior change is a process with five stages.

1. Pre-contemplation happens before you start thinking about change.

2. Contemplation is the process of considering making a change within the next six months.

3. Preparation is when you are getting things in order so that you can make a change within the next month.

4. Action is the doing it phase. You are actually putting your plans and preparation into effect.

5. Maintenance means the change is becoming a normal part of your life.

☞ Failure is part of the process. You can expect to have lapses or "fall off the wagon." The key is to learn from your mistakes and start again.

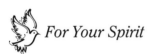 *For Your Spirit*

Taking the Lead

You must have a really powerful personality if you know how to get 12 guys to quit their jobs and leave their families to embark on an uncertain journey to change the world. If collecting followers is a hallmark of leadership, then Jesus is almost certainly the greatest leader in history. Of course his leadership ability was ordained and anointed by a Higher Power, but that doesn't mean he didn't have some practical leadership skills, too.

Jesus was wise, encouraging, and generally gentle, but he could get tough with folks if necessary. He gave clear instructions and he earned people's faith and trust. He knew how to command large crowds and advise people one-on-one. He made himself "one of us" and spoke to people on their own level in their own terms. All of these qualities made Him a model of spiritual leadership—for his apostles and followers in his day, and for generations of church leaders, business executives, and regular people like us.

Leadership doesn't just apply to guiding other people. Leadership also applies to our own self direction. The same clarity, encouragement, and wisdom that we would ideally use in leading others, we should also apply to our own lives. This self direction is an important part of taking care of your health.

Your doctor or other healthcare providers can give you direction; that's what they're there for. But ultimately you have to be able to direct your own path and find your own way. There will be moments when you have to make a decision on your own. Early in the morning, the doctor won't be available to tell you to get out of bed and go for your daily jog. When it's midnight and you know there's a half-gallon of ice cream in the freezer, there's no nutritionist to advise you to eat some fruit instead. You're the boss. You decide.

Some great leaders are born that way. Others of us have to work on developing our leadership skills. Especially when it comes to how we treat ourselves. Too often we beat ourselves up for our failures or we don't encourage ourselves to meet goals—things we wouldn't do to someone else.

Ultimately leadership comes from within. Spending time in contemplation and preparing yourself at the soul level can help you make wise choices—even if you're just standing in front of the freezer looking at that carton of ice cream. And as you take positive action and see yourself making healthy choices through a period of time, you are further developing your confidence in your ability to lead. It is a quality that will serve you well in all aspects of your own life, and make you able to serve others in valuable ways.

5 NUTRITION BUILDING BLOCKS

When you got your diabetes diagnosis, what was the first thing you thought? For many people, the first thing that comes to mind is: *What will I be able to eat?* That's because back in the day, people talked about diabetes in terms of what you *couldn't* eat. No bread. No dessert. Avoid all forms of sugar or anything that might turn to sugar—at least that's what people said.

It's true that diabetes has a closer association with food than perhaps any other disease. And what you eat has a big impact on how well you can manage the disease. But having diabetes doesn't mean the end of good eating. The principles of a healthy diet are the same for the person with diabetes as they are for everyone else. If you eat wisely and well, you can still enjoy delicious food despite your disease. Even if you eat traditional soul, Caribbean, or Creole food, you'll be happy to know that many traditional dishes can stay on your grocery list. No kidding.

You won't have to miss out on a big pot of beans or black-eyed peas. You can still make collards or turnip greens. Even sweet potatoes and corn bread can stay on your menu.

Foods like these are high in fiber, vitamins, and minerals and, depending on how you cook them, low in fat. Yes, creating diabetes-friendly meals may require eating a little less of this and more of that. But the bottom line is you need to eat a variety of foods to get all the nutrients you body needs for good health—and that's true whether you have diabetes or not. The food you eat should provide the right balance of carbohydrates, protein, fat, vitamins, minerals, fiber, and water. All of these nutrients working together give you the energy you need for a full and productive lifestyle.

If one thing is going to change about how you eat, it's the ability to eat whatever, whenever. As a person with diabetes, you have to pay more careful attention to the way you balance your diet. The key to eating well—and managing your blood sugar—lies in how you mix and match the nutrition essentials. In this chapter we're going to get a good grasp on the elements of an ideal diet. And then we're going to learn how to put them together into delicious and diabetes-appropriate meals.

Carbohydrates

If your body could choose one source of energy, it would choose carbs. Contrary to what many of the popular fad diets will tell you, your body *needs* carbohydrates. In fact, carbohydrates, at 4 calories per gram, should make up 45 to 60 percent of your daily calories.

Now, you're probably saying, "I thought carbohydrates were bad for people with diabetes." No, carbohydrates are not bad. But if you eat too many of them at a meal or snack, they will cause your blood glucose level to go up higher than you want. In the next chapter, you'll learn how you can successfully make carbs part of your daily meal plan. For now, just breath a sigh of relief: you can still eat a hot roll once in a while.

The three main types of carbohydrates are sugar, starch, and fiber.

If I say **sugar**, you probably first think of that sparkly white stuff in the covered bowl on your breakfast table. But sugar is called by many names—simple sugar, table sugar, cane sugar, brown sugar, turbinado, demerara. maple syrup, molasses, honey, and high-fructose corn syrup—they're all sugars. And fructose and lactose? Yep, sugar from fruit and milk respectively. Medical types may call it fast-acting carbohydrate, but it's still just sugar. The main differences is that the naturally occurring sugar in some foods comes with many nutritional benefits like the fiber in fruit, the calcium in milk, and the iron in molasses. When you start adding sugar to foods though, you're not increasing the nutritional value, just boosting calories (and these processed foods tend to have added fat as well). But once any kind of sugar hits your belly, your body can't tell the difference between sugars that are in foods naturally or those that are added to foods. It's all just sugar that turns to glucose in your bloodstream.

Starch, the second type of carbohydrate, is also basically sugar. It's made from sugar molecules that are linked together in long chains. High-starch foods include bread, cereal, pasta, crackers, starchy vegetables (green peas, corn, lima beans, potatoes), and dried beans (pinto beans, kidney beans, black-eyed peas, and split peas). During digestion, starches are broken down and converted to glucose.

Fiber is the third type of carbohydrate. Fiber is the indigestible part of any plant food, including the leaves of vegetables, fruit skins, and seeds.

If you eat a fibrous food—even one with sugar (say, an apple) or starch (whole grain bread)—the fiber slows the conversion of the sugar or starch into glucose, keeping the blood sugar more stable. Because fiber can't be digested completely, it adds bulk and helps to move food waste out of the body more quickly.

A good source of fiber contains 3 to 5 grams per serving. Some good sources of fiber are:

> Whole-grain products, including breads from whole wheat, rye, bran, oat, and corn flour or cornmeal; pastas; whole-grain or bran cereals; brown rice.

> Vegetables such as broccoli, brussels sprouts, cabbage, carrots and green peas; lentils, dried beans, and peas; sweet potatoes, turnips, and other root vegetables; and all forms of leafy greens—cooked or raw.

> Fruits including apples, bananas, berries, cantaloupes, kiwi, oranges, peaches, grapes, pears, and melons. Also, dried fruits, such as raisins and dried apricots.

> Nuts (peanuts, walnuts, almonds) and seeds (sesame, sunflower, pumpkin).

Ultimately, it's the total number of carbs—sugar, starch, or fiber—that matters in your meal, not the type of carbohydrate. If you balance sugars, starchy food, and fiber in your meals for an ideal number of carbs, you can enjoy a healthy, delectable meal.

Nutrition Guidelines for Carbohydrates and Diabetes

> Food containing carbohydrates from whole grains, fruits, vegetables, and low-fat milk should be included in a healthy diet.

> The total amount of carbohydrates in meals and snacks is more important than the source or type.

> Sugar counts as a carbohydrate sources in a meal, but low-calorie sweeteners don't have to be counted as carbs in your meal plan.

> 45 to 60 percent of the total calories you eat each day should come from carbohydrates.

> A healthy fiber intake is 20 to 35 grams daily or 14 grams per 1,000 calories.

The Sweet Life

There are plenty of sweet foods out there that don't actually have sugar in them. These are foods manufactured with nonnutritive sweeteners—reduced-calorie, low-calorie, and no-calorie sugar substitutes. These sweeteners are created from alcohols, amino acids, and other chemical formulas that have been approved by the Food and Drug Administration (FDA) for dietary use.

Sugar Alcohols also referred to as polyols are one type of reduced-calorie sweetener. They have about 2 calories per gram—half the calories of table sugar. Contrary to their name, polyols are not sugar or alcohol the way we think of them. When you're reading labels, you'll recognize them easily because their names always end in "ol"—sorbitol, xylitol, erythritol, maltitol, mannitol. Keep an eye out for these because they should be used in moderation. Using large amounts of sorbitol (more than 50 grams a day) or mannitol (more than 20 grams a day) can cause diarrhea and upset stomach.

Low-calorie sweeteners are also known as sugar substitutes. They provide practically no calories and won't increase your blood-glucose levels. There are lots of them on the market these days—in prepared foods, in food and drink mixes, and packaged to be added to food like sugar. Common sugar substitutes include:

- *Aspartame.* A combination of the amino acids phenylalanine and aspartic acid, it's 220 times sweeter than sugar. Brand names are NutraSweet, Equal, and NutraTaste, and you'll find it in low-calorie beverages and dry drink mixes, chewing gum, candy, gelatins, dessert mixes, puddings and fillings, frozen desserts, and yogurt. People with phenylketonuria (PKU), a rare genetic condition that affects metabolism, should not use aspartame.
- *Acesulfame K,* also called acesulfame potassium or ace-K, is 200 times sweeter than sugar. Packaged under the brand names Sweet One, Sunette, and Swiss Sweet, it's used in cooking, baking, and as a table top sweetener, and it can be found in desserts, puddings, soft drinks, candies, and canned foods.
- *Saccharin* has been used as a no-calorie sweetener for over 100 years, most popularly in little pink packets of Sweet 'n Low.

Three hundred times sweeter than sugar, saccharin can be found in sugar-free foods and beverages including baked goods, jams, chewing gum, canned fruit, candy, dessert toppings and salad dressing. Its other brand names are Sugar Twin and Necta Sweet. The ADI for saccharin is 5 mg/kg body weight per day. A 150 pound person can safely consume 8½ packets every day.

- **Sucralose** is made from sugar but is 600 times sweeter than sugar. Sucralose, brand named Splenda can be found in a broad range of foods, beverages and table top sweeteners.

- **Neotame** is the newest food ingredient that can be used as a sweetener and flavor enhancer, and it's a whopping 8,000 times sweeter than sugar. You'll find it in baked goods, soft drinks, chewing gum, frosting, frozen desserts, jams and jellies, gelatins, puddings, processed fruit and fruit juices, and syrups. It can be used alone or blended with other non-nutritive or nutritive sweeteners.

- **Rebiana** is the name for rebaudioside A, an extract from the leaves of the stevia plant. It's 200 times sweeter than table sugar and can be found in a variety of foods and beverages and in tabletop sweeteners under the brand names Truvia and PureVia.

⁓

Sugar Substitute Safety

Some years ago, saccharin and other artificial sweeteners were linked with cancer, causing quite a scare among diabetes patients who had come to rely on the little pink packets to sweeten their coffee and tea. Researchers went into overdrive trying to determine whether the experiments that caused cancer in lab rats actually translated into human health. They found no definitive connection. The National Cancer Institute issued an official statement that rules out any connection between artificial sweeteners and cancers. For details, go to *www.cancer.gov*.

Even so, there are limits on how much of a given artificial sweetener a person should consume each day. In most cases, it's far more than a person would want or need, but it's helpful to keep track of how much you're consuming. Here's a way to look at it.

Sugar Sub	Acceptable daily intake (ADI)	=	Equivalent for 150-pound person
Aspartame	50 mg/kg of body weight	=	15 cans of soda
Acesulfame K	15 mg/kg of body weight	=	25 cans of soda
Saccharin	5 mg/kg of body weight	=	8 ½ packets
Sucralose	5 mg/kg of body weight	=	5 cans of soda
Neotame	2 mg/kg of body weight	=	22 cans of soda
Rebiana	12 mg/kg of body weight	=	24 8 oz. servings of soda

Just because artificial sweeteners have been pronounced safe and they have the benefit of not affecting your glucose, doesn't mean that you *have* to use sugar substitutes in great quantities—or at all. If you'd rather go the natural sweetener route—or if you just don't like the taste of faux sugar, you can work nutritive sweeteners into your diet. Just work closely with your dream team, keep a careful eye on your blood sugar and balance your diet carefully.

Protein

Protein can be found in every cell of the body. Your organs, muscles, nervous system, blood vessels, and skeleton are all made of and dependent on protein. It is used to build and repair body tissue and keep your hair, nails, and skin healthy. It also helps to boost your immune system. Like carbs, protein provides energy for the body; however, it is not the body's preferred energy source. The body likes to use protein primarily to repair those tissues. It won't use protein as an energy source unless no carbs are available. Each gram of protein contains 4 calories.

Protein is made up of building blocks called amino acids. There are 20 different amino acids; nine of them are considered essential, because the body can't make them on its own. These must come from the food you eat—both plant and animal food sources.

Protein from animals—meat, fish, dairy, and eggs—contains all nine essential amino acids and is considered a "complete" protein. Soy is the only plant food that can make that claim. Grains, legumes, nuts, and seeds are good sources of plant protein, but these and other plant foods don't contain enough of one or more of the essential amino acids—each one is missing something. It's only by eating a wide variety of plant protein during the course of a day that you get all of the essential amino acids. However, plant foods have the advantage of not having the fat and cholesterol that animal products do. So again, balancing the proteins in your diet is as important as balancing the carbohydrates.

Nutrition Guidelines for Protein and Diabetes

▶ Approximately 15 to 20 percent of total calories should come from protein.

▶ Choose protein sources that are low in saturated fat and cholesterol, such as poultry, fish, legumes, beans (soy, pinto, black, and kidney), grains, nuts, low-fat dairy, and egg whites.

▶ It is not necessary to have a protein source at each meal. Try to get about 5 to 7 ounces of protein in a day.

▶ If you have well-controlled type 2 diabetes, protein will not cause a rise in your blood glucose levels.

Fat and Cholesterol

Though "fat" seems to be a bad word in our society, fat plays an important role in our health. Fat is the most concentrated source of energy for the body—providing nine calories per gram, more than twice the amount of energy found in carbohydrates and protein. The body stores energy in the form of fat, and fat is essential to insulate the body tissues, protect the vital organs, and transport and absorb the fat-soluble vitamins A, D, E, and K. And when it comes to food, fat is undeniable in its ability to make food taste good—enhancing food flavor, making baked products tender, and providing a smooth, silky feeling in the mouth. So fat itself isn't "bad"—depending on how much and what kind you consume.

Fats—a term that includes oils, butter, margarine, lard, and other fats found in animal foods—are made up of fatty acids that are linked together. There are three types of fatty acids— saturated, monounsaturated, and polyunsaturated—and all fats and oils are made up of a combination of the three. The predominant type of fat in a food determines which category the food falls into. However it is important to remember that when it comes to calories, "fat is fat," and all types provide 9 calories per gram.

Saturated fatty acids are usually solid at room temperature and are found mostly in foods that come from animals, such as meat, lard, bacon, poultry, dairy products, butterfat, and eggs. But coconut oil, palm kernel oil, and palm oil are also saturated fats. This type of fat can cause your body to produce too much cholesterol.

Monounsaturated fatty acids are usually liquid at room temperature and are found mostly in vegetable oils such as canola, olive, and peanut oils, and in whole olives and peanuts. Monounsaturated fats are often called heart-healthy fats because they don't cause increased cholesterol level.

Polyunsaturated fatty acids are usually liquid or soft at room temperature and are found mostly in vegetable oils such as safflower, sunflower, corn, and flaxseed. Salmon, albacore tuna, herring, and mackerel are called "fatty fish" because they contain a form of polyunsaturated fatty acid called omega-3. Omega-3 is thought to help lower levels of triglycerides, the form of fat that is stored in the body. Walnuts are also a good source of omega-3 fatty acids.

Just as there are essential amino acids, there are essential fatty acids—those the body needs for cell structure and hormone formation. Linoleic acid and alpha-linolenic acid are the two essential polyunsaturated fatty acids that must be obtained from food. You get linoleic acid in vegetable oils such as soybean, corn, and safflower oil. Alpha-linolenic acid is found mostly in fatty fish.

Trans-fatty acids are polyunsaturated fats that have been chemically changed to make them stay solid at room temperature. Hydrogenated vegetable oils such as vegetable shortening and margarine contain trans-fatty acids—as do the foods you make with these oils. Trans fatty acids may act as saturated fat in the body, raising your cholesterol levels. If you're looking out for the foods that contain the most trans fats, check baked foods such as cakes, cookies, pies, and breads. And watch the margarine you spread on your toast.

Cholesterol is another dirty word in the world of nutrition, but in fact it's something the body makes because the body needs it—at least a little. This waxy substance, found in the blood, is manufactured in your liver to build cell membranes and brain and nerve tissue. It helps the body form hormones needed to regulate the body and helps create bile acids you need for digestion. Any additional cholesterol that winds up in the bloodstream comes from animal foods you eat such as egg yolks, meat (especially organ meats like liver), and full-fat dairy products like milk and cheese.

Cholesterol is carried in the bloodstream in "packages" of fat and protein called lipoprotein. But not all cholesterol is the same and the different kinds behave differently in the body. That's why your cholesterol test results itemize HDL and LDL cholesterol. LDL or low-density lipoprotein is the "bad" cholesterol. Too much of it can increase the risk of heart disease, because it causes fatty deposits to form in the arteries. Cholesterol carried in packages called high-density lipoproteins (HDL) cholesterol is the "good" stuff. HDL cholesterol seems to protect against heart disease, because it helps to remove excess cholesterol from the blood and carry it to the liver, where it can be excreted.

```
┌─────────────────────────────────────────────────────────────────────┐
│                    Cholesterol and Fat Goals                        │
│                                                                     │
│  HDL cholesterol          over 40 mg/dL* for men;                   │
│                           over 50 mg/dL for women                   │
│  LDL cholesterol          under 100 mg/dL;  under 70 mg/dL for high risk individuals │
│  **Triglycerides          under 150 mg/dL                           │
│  Total cholesterol        under 200 mg/dL                           │
│                                                                     │
│  *mg/dL stands for milligrams per deciliter, a volume measure of blood. │
│  **Triglycerides are the storage form of fat.                       │
└─────────────────────────────────────────────────────────────────────┘
```

Nutrition Guidelines for Fat and Cholesterol and Diabetes

▸ Limit total daily calories from fat to 20 to 30 percent.

▸ Get only 7 to 10 percent of your total daily calories from saturated fat

▸ Keep total trans-fat intake as low as possible—about 1 to 3 grams daily

▸ Consume less than 300 mg cholesterol daily.

▸ Choose low-fat and reduced-calorie foods wisely, because they can contain more carbohydrate than the full-fat food.

▸ Consume 3 to 4 servings of fish weekly, including fatty fish such as salmon and tuna.

▸ Avoid organ meats like liver.

Water

Most people don't include water in conversations about nutrients. We just don't think of it the way we think of our vitamins and minerals—as essential for our body's growth and development. As a result, most people fail to meet their daily water requirements.

But in reality, water is as much a nutrient as iron or Vitamin C. We need it to help digest food, carry waste from the cells, and control body temperature. Water in our bloodstream metabolizes and transports the carbohydrates and proteins that our bodies use as food.

Although about 60 percent of the human body is composed of water, the Institute of Medicine recommends that women consume 11 cups of fluid per day; men should have 16 cups of fluid daily to stay fully hydrated. About 80 percent of your daily fluid intake should come from water and other beverages that you drink. The other 20 percent can come from juicy foods like fruits and vegetables.

Vitamins and Minerals

Vitamins are needed for normal growth and development of the body. Vitamins don't provide energy, as some folks commonly believe, but they do help the body break down carbohydrates, protein, and fat, and use them more efficiently. The body requires very small quantities of vitamins, but it cannot function properly without them.

Vitamins fit into two basic classifications: water-soluble and fat-soluble.

Water-soluble vitamins are those that are flushed away when we eliminate water from out bodies. Because they can't be stored, you have to replace them in the body daily. The water-soluble vitamins are B and C.

You don't lose **fat-soluble vitamins** every day. These vitamins, including A, D, E, and K, are stored in the liver and fat tissue of the body and dispensed as needed. But because you can't flush them out easily, fat-soluble vitamins can be toxic if you take them in large quantities. The "Daily Vitamin and Mineral Guide" on pages 67–70 can tell you how much is enough and how much is too much of any given vitamin.

There is no clear evidence that a person with diabetes gets any extra benefit from vitamin supplements unless she already has a vitamin or mineral deficiency. In other words, a vitamin isn't going to help you control your diabetes. But there's no harm in using a vitamin or mineral supplement as a nutritional backup. Just make sure you discuss it with your doctor or health-care provider first. Many supplements contain active ingredients that have strong biological effects, and they're not always safe for every user. Other supplements may interact with prescription and over-the-counter medicines. Taking these products without medical supervision may put you at risk.

Sound Advice

Turn on the TV and flip channels for a while. Eventually, you're going to come across some "breaking news" about a new formula or supplement "clinically proven" to normalize your blood sugar and reverse diabetes. Think about this for a moment—a cure for diabetes in a bottle? Oh, if it were only that simple. Yet, that's what the companies that market such products want you to believe. The TV pitch is so great, you think to yourself, "It should work. It was clinically proven, right?" Wrong! The claims are nothing more than great marketing techniques used to gain your trust. If there were something that would reverse diabetes, it would make every headline in America, not just the late-night infomercial circuit.

Daily Vitamin and Mineral Guide

	Function	Food Source	Recommended Dietary Allowance	Tolerable upper intake level/ adverse effects
Vitamin A	Normal vision, growth development, and reproduction. Healthy skin, teeth, and bones. Also helps fight infection and prevents cell destruction.	Liver, dairy products, fish, dark-colored fruits and leafy vegetables, collards, kale, carrots, mango, plantain, pumpkin, sweet potato.	700 mcg/day for women (2300 IU). 900 mcg/day for men (3,000 IU).	3,000 mcg/day (10,000 IU). Hair loss, rash, mouth sores and liver toxicity.
Vitamin B6 (Pyridoxine)	Normal growth. Also participates in metabolism of protein and carbohydrates.	Fortified cereals, organ meats, fortified soy-based meat substitutes, spinach, bananas.	Under 50: 1.3 mg/day. Women over 50: 1.5 mg/day. Men over 50: 1.7 mg/day.	100 mg/day. Over 200 mg/day can lead to sensory neuropathy.
Vitamin B12 (Cobalamin)	Keeps red blood cells and the nervous system healthy; participates in energy metabolism.	Fortified cereals, meat, fish, poultry, dairy, liver, and kidney.	2.4 mcg/day.	Not determined.
Folic Acid/ Folate	Prevents birth defects. Participates in formation of red blood cells, metabolism of protein, and normal digestive system functions.	Enriched cereal grains, dark leafy vegetables, enriched and whole-grain breads and bread products, fortified ready-to-eat cereals, black-eyed-peas, pinto and navy beans, spinach, collard greens, kidney, liver.	400 mcg/day.	1,000 mcg/day. Upper limit applies to synthetic forms obtained from supplements and/or fortified foods.

	Function	Food Source	Recommended Dietary Allowance	Tolerable upper intake level/ adverse effects
Niacin (B3)	Helps release energy, promotes good physical and mental health, healthy skin, tongue, and digestive system.	Meat, fish, poultry, enriched and whole-grain breads and bread products, fortified ready-to-eat cereals, peanuts, tomato products, beef liver.	14 mg/day for women; 16 mg/day for men.	35 mg/day. Upper limit applies to synthetic forms obtained from supplements and/or fortified foods. High levels associated with flushing, high blood glucose, and liver damage.
Riboflavin (B2)	Helps release energy. Promotes growth and cellular metabolism, healthy eyes, skin, lips, and tongue.	Organ meats, milk, dairy products, fortified cereals and bread products, almonds, eggs, and fish.	1.1 mg/day for women; 1.3 mg/day for men.	Not determined.
Thiamin (B1)	Participates in the metabolism of carbohydrates and protein.	Enriched, fortified, or whole-grain products, bread and bread products, grain, beef liver, almonds, fish, spinach, lima beans, and corn.	1.1 mg/day for women; 1.3 mg/day for men.	Not determined.
Vitamin C	Helps maintain body tissue and promote wound healing. Protects the body against infection and oxidative destruction.	Citrus fruits, tomatoes, tomato juice, potatoes, brussels sprouts, cauliflower, broccoli, guava, strawberries, orange juice, papaya, peppers.	75 mg/day for women; 90 mg/day for men.	2,000 mg/day. Diarrhea and other gastrointestinal disturbances and increase the risk of kidney stones.

	Function	Food Source	Recommended Dietary Allowance	Tolerable upper intake level/ adverse effects
Vitamin D	Helps maintain normal blood levels of calcium and phosphorus, aids in the absorption of calcium, helping to form and maintain strong bones.	Fish, eggs, fortified milk, and cod liver oil.	5 mcg (200 IU). If you are 50-70 yrs old, you need 10 mcg/day; 70+ need15 mcg/ day (600 IU).	2,000 IU/day. Excess calcium in the blood and excess bone loss.
Vitamin E	Prevents destruction of cell membranes.	Vegetable oils, unprocessed cereal grains, nuts, fruits, vegetables, meats, sunflower seeds, almonds, spinach, tomato.	15 mg/day as tocopherol.	1,000 mg/day. Hemorrhage.
Vitamin K	Necessary for normal clotting of blood.	Green, leafy vegetables such as spinach, broccoli, asparagus, watercress, cabbage, cauliflower, green peas, beans, olives, canola, soybeans, meat, cereals, and dairy products.	90 mcg/day for women; 120 mcg/day for men.	Not determined. Blood clots, break down of red blood cells and jaundice.
Calcium	Essential role in blood clotting, muscle contraction, blood pressure, nerve transmission, and bone and tooth formation.	Milk, cheese, yogurt, corn tortillas, calcium-set tofu, Chinese cabbage, kale, broccoli and brussels sprouts.	1,000 mg/day for adults under 50; 1,200 mg/day for adults over 50 years.	2,500 mg/day. Kidney stones, increased blood calcium, and renal insufficiency.

	Function	Food Source	Recommended Dietary Allowance	Tolerable upper intake level/ adverse effects
Chromium	Enhances the action of insulin, helps maintain normal blood glucose levels.	Some cereals, meats, poultry, fish, beer, brewer's yeast, cheese, broccoli, beans, seeds, wine.	No RDA set adequate intake. 25 mcg/day women 50+ 20 mcg/day. Men 35 mcg/day men 50+ 30 mcg/ day.	Not determined. Chronic renal failure associated with excessive consumption.
Iron	Essential for red blood cell formation.	Fruits, vegetables, meat, poultry, and fortified bread and grain products such as cereal, navy, kidney and lima beans, collards, and nuts.	18 mg/day for premenopausal women; 8mg/ day for men and postmenopausal women.	45 mg/day. Gastrointestinal disturbances, nausea, vomiting, constipation, or diarrhea.
Magnesium	Participates in enzyme systems, assists in calcium and potassium uptake.	Green leafy vegetables, nuts, fish, milk, brown rice, and baked potato with skin.	320 mg/day for women, 420 mg/ day for men.	350 mg/day. Supplements containing magnesium may cause diarrhea.
Selenium	Defends against oxidative stress; regulates thyroid hormone actions.	Organ meats, seafood, whole grains, nuts, and sunflower seeds.	55 mcg/day.	400 mcg/day. Hair and nail brittleness and loss.
Vanadium	Biological function in humans is not fully understood.	Mushrooms, shellfish, black pepper, parsley, and dill seed.	No RDA or adequate intake established.	1.8 mg/day. Renal dysfunction.
Zinc	Protein synthesis, taste sensitivity, and cell growth.	Fortified cereals, red meats, seafood, eggs, beans and peas.	8 mg/day for women, 11 mg/day for men.	40 mg/day. Interference with the absorption of copper.

How do you know that what you are reading or hearing is sound advice? Unfortunately, the current rules and regulations make it a little difficult to tell whether something is good for you or just marketed that way. The Federal Food, Drug, and Cosmetic Act is the law that regulates foods and prescription medications. It requires the Food and Drug Administration (FDA) to approve prescription and over-the-counter drugs before companies can market them in the United States. The FDA is very strict in how it evaluates these drugs.

Supplements, however, are a different story. Under the Dietary Supplement Health and Education Act (DSHEA), companies can market supplements as long as they use "truthful and non-misleading claims." The companies can't claim or imply that a supplement can "prevent, diagnose, mitigate, treat, or cure a disease." If it could do any of these things, it would classify as a drug and need to have FDA approval.

But the FDA process takes time and costs money. So what do companies do? They word the description of their product ambiguously ("This product supports diabetes health."). And the DSHEA requires that they contain a disclaimer that reads, "This statement has not been evaluated by the Food and Drug Administration. This product is not intended to diagnose, treat, cure, or prevent any disease." This disclaimer tells you that if the supplement claims to cure an illness, the FDA has not tested this supplement for safety and effectiveness.

Then there are the claims that certain foods or drinks regulate diabetes. Food claims are even harder to evaluate; they're not regulated and they don't need to contain this disclaimer.

The best way to know whether a claim made about a supplement or food is true, is to understand the difference between claims:

▶ Solid health claims are claims based on scientific evidence and approved by the FDA. These trustworthy claims will name a disease such as cancer, stroke, or heart disease, and usually refer to a diet that is low (or high) in some nutrient. An example of this type of claim can be found on Quaker oatmeal containers: "Three grams of soluble fiber daily from oatmeal, in a diet low in saturated fat and cholesterol, may reduce the risk of heart disease. This cereal has two grams per serving."

▶ Preliminary health claims are based on incomplete evidence. A study may have been done, but not corroborated or supported enough to earn FDA approval. These claims must contain a disclaimer such as, "the FDA has determined that this evidence is limited and not conclusive" or "the FDA concludes that there is little scientific evidence supporting this claim."

▶ Structure or function claims require no prior approval by the FDA. This makes the claims highly doubtful. There might not be scientific research that backs up the claim or the supporting research may have been poor or incomplete. Look for words such as "maintains," "supports," or "enhances." An example of a structure or function claim might read "keeps your blood-sugar function on the right track."

Power Points

🖙 People with diabetes can eat just about anything they want—if they are aware of how it will affect their blood sugar.

🖙 Carbs are an important nutrition building block—even for people with diabetes. Between 45 and 60 percent of your diet should be high-fiber, whole grain, and nutrient-dense carbs. Sugar and other refined carbs can cause blood glucose to spike.

🖙 Proteins should make up 15 to 20 percent of your diet. Complete proteins are found in animal foods and soy products. You can get enough protein from plant foods by eating a wide variety of them.

🖙 All fats aren't bad for you. Monounsaturated fat doesn't increase cholesterol levels; polyunsaturated omega-3 fats reduce triglyceride levels. Avoid trans fats and saturated fats.

🖙 The body makes the cholesterol it needs. A high level of HDL cholesterol protects against heart disease. LDL cholesterol increases the risk of heart disease.

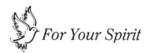 *For Your Spirit*

Going to the Rock

Using the term "building blocks" may seem like a strange metaphor to describe food and nutrition. But we use the term because nutrition is the basis for good health—especially if you have diabetes. Managing your condition relies on your ability to eat healthfully, mindfully, and well. It is indeed the foundation for your diabetes care. If you don't eat well, all the medicine in the world won't be able to help you.

It's important to have a firm foundation for any important endeavor—whether it is in starting a new health program or beginning any new, important venture in your life. If you start a new job, you want to do so on the foundation of good training and experience. If you're about to commit to a love relationship, you want it built on a solid foundation of care and respect. The same goes for beginning a new health regimen: you want to do it based on the best information available and the strongest support system possible. Establishing a firm foundation gives you a good base from which to make sound health decisions later. If your foundation is unsteady, you won't have the confidence and sense of security that will sustain you as you try to maintain your health or build on your efforts.

In our churches, we often hear people talking and singing about "going to the Rock." That "Rock" is the foundation of their faith—the thing that they *know* with all their heart they can rely on. Keeping that connection with the rock is probably the very reason people go to church at all. And it's vital to your mental and spiritual well-being to feel anchored and secure in your world. You have to have a rock.

Whether we're talking on the spiritual realm or the physical realm, you must have a rock—something you are certain you can depend on to hold you up and pull you through. If you know you can depend on your best friend or a family member to have your back as you walk this path with diabetes, you are very fortunate. Praise and appreciate the people (and circumstances) that offer you that unwavering support.

But also know that, ultimately, you will find your rock within you. It may be your faith. It may be your sense of determination—that no matter what happens you are committed to doing the thing you say you are going to do. Ironically, your rock may be your flexibility—your ability to flow with whatever life presents to you and make the best of it. But know that you have a God-given *something* within you that will sustain you when no one else can. It is this rock and your faith in it, that will carry you through this health journey—and the long journey that is your life.

6 Building a Diabetes Pyramid

When you were first diagnosed with diabetes, you probably received information about medications and glucose monitoring, as well as some very vague instruction on meal planning: "Stay away from sugar," "Lose some weight," "Don't eat fat," "Eat smaller portions." Sound familiar? Good advice, certainly, but so vague. Carefully planning your meals and changing you eating behavior are the most difficult aspects of diabetes self-management. It's a whole lot more than just "avoiding sugar." The good news is that you can manage diabetes successfully if you have the proper meal-planning strategies.

In the early days of diabetes care, patients were put on carefully restricted diets that limited starches and sweets. But in 1994 the American Diabetes Association announced that there is no longer a universal "diabetic diet." Instead there are tools that can be used—based on your individual health assessment—to help achieve your diabetes goals. That opened the way for folks to develop different kinds of strategies to successfully control diabetes. This chapter looks at one of the most popular meal plans: the diabetes food guide pyramid and a variation of it that focuses on ethnic food. In the next chapter, we will examine carbohydrate counting and the glycemic index counting method of making meal plans.

The Diabetes Food Pyramid

The **Food Guide Pyramid** was released by the U.S. Department of Agriculture (USDA) in 1992. It was designed to graphically illustrate the Dietary Guidelines for Americans which were established to promote good health among U.S. citizens. Foods in the lower, wider section of the pyramid are the foods that should be eaten more often and in the largest amounts—fruits, vegetables, and grains. Meat and dairy products fall midway of the pyramid; and fats, oils and sweets are in the point at the very top, indicating that they should be eaten less often and in smaller amounts.

In 2005, the USDA replaced its familiar pyramid with **MyPyramid**, emphasizing the need for a more individualized approach to improving diet and lifestyle. It represents the recommended proportion of foods from each food group, and focuses on the importance of making smart food choices in every food group.

Then there's the **Diabetes Food Pyramid.** It was developed to offer an individualized approach to improving diet and lifestyle. The Diabetes Food Pyramid looks a lot like the original Food Guide Pyramid but groups foods based on their carbohydrate and protein content, rather than their food classification. For example, you will find black-eyed peas and sweet potatoes in the grain group instead of the vegetable group. Cheese will be found in the meat group instead of the milk group.

The portion sizes are a little different too. They changed so that each serving of carbohydrate-containing food has the same carb content—about 15 grams. In the Diabetes Food Pyramid a serving of vegetables is 1 1/2 cup, a serving of rice or pasta is 1/3 cup and a serving of fruit juice is 1/2 cup.

You'll notice that the diabetes pyramid doesn't tell you how many servings of food to eat a day. That's because the number of servings depends on your weight, activity level, health goals, and the foods you like to eat. A chart gives you specifics a little later in the chapter.

This pyramid was helpful to diabetes patients in general, but I found that my clients from down south, the Caribbean and Africa had trouble figuring out where their traditional foods fit in the pyramid. Are stewed tomatoes still a vegetable? Where does peanut stew fit in? I developed the **Diabetes Soul Food Pyramid** to offer African-Americans and anyone who loves "soul food," an individualized approach to improving diet and lifestyle. The key message of the Diabetes Soul Food Pyramid is that you don't have to give up ethnic food, but simply learn how to place it in your diet successfully.

A little later, you'll learn to design your own pyramid—one that you can modify as your goals and health needs change. For now, let's examine each food group along with tips for healthy food preparation and selection. (Check the back of the book for a more extensive listing of foods from each category of the pyramid. If you like Caribbean, Cajun, or Creole cuisine you will find your favorites included. You will also find a two-week sample menu.)

Diabetes Soul Food Pyramid

```
                        Fat
                      0 grams
                    carboyhydrate

              Milk        │  Fish, Poultry,
                          │    and Meat
            15 grams      │    0 grams
          carboyhydrate   │  carboyhydrate

        Vegetables        │        Fruits
    15 grams carboyhydrate │  15 grams carboyhydrate

              Starch/Grains
           15 grams carboyhydrate
```

Starch Group

As you'd expect, the starch group includes bagels, bread, muffins, cereals, crackers, and noodles. But it might surprise you to see that it also includes starchy vegetables and root veggies such as corn, peas, white and sweet potatoes, and all kinds of beans.

Breads, Rice, Grains, and Pasta

▸ Eat at least three ounces of whole grain products per day. (One ounce is about 1 slice of bread or about 1 cup of ready-to-eat breakfast cereal.)

▸ Make at least half of the grains you eat whole grains, such as brown rice, buckwheat, bulgur, oatmeal, wild rice, and whole-wheat bread, crackers, pasta, and tortillas.

▸ Eat fewer fried and high-fat starches, such as biscuits, corn bread, dressing/stuffing, pancakes, or waffles.

▸ Limit additional butter, margarine, mayonnaise, shortening, and oil.

▸ Add vegetables, such as onions and peppers, to rice instead of additional fat and oil.

▸ Eat brown rice instead of white rice.

▶ Check the ingredient list on grain product labels. For whole-grain products, you will see the words "whole" or "whole-grain" before the grain ingredient's name.

    ▷ Replace half the white flour in recipes with whole-wheat flour.

    ▷ Use oatmeal, bran, or whole-wheat flour to make muffins.

    ▷ When making cornbread use whole cornmeal.

▶ Use whole-wheat pasta when making pasta salad, macaroni-and-cheese, and other pasta dishes.

    ▷ Check the Nutrition Facts label for the fiber content of food products. Fiber content is a good clue to the amount of whole grain in the product.

Beans

▶ Canned beans of all types are packed with fiber, protein, and antioxidants.

▶ If you use canned beans make sure the label says "no salt added" or "low-sodium." Rinse them before you cook them to reduce the sodium content.

▶ Cook beans with smoked turkey instead of salt pork, ham hocks, neck bones, or fatback.

Starchy Vegetables

▶ Instead of frying starchy vegetables try boiling, steaming, or baking them. Corn, peas, potatoes, sweet potatoes, winter squash, and yams are all starchy vegetables.

▶ Add less sugar to sweet potatoes and yams. Try using a sugar substitute that is made for cooking and baking.

▶ Season starchy vegetables with onions, garlic, peppers, and herbs instead of salt and fat.

Vegetable Group

Any vegetable or 100-percent vegetable juice counts as a member of the vegetable group. Fresh, frozen, and canned veggies all count the same toward meeting vegetable intake goals.

▶ Eat raw and cooked vegetables with little or no fat.

    ▷ If you do use a small amount of fat, use canola, olive oil, or tub margarine instead of fat from meat, butter, or shortening.

- ▶ Steam vegetables using a small amount of water or low-fat broth.
- ▶ For canned vegetables, "no salt added" is the best choice.
- ▶ Mix in some chopped onion or garlic for added flavor, or use a little vinegar, or lemon or lime juice.
  - ▷ Cook vegetables with smoked turkey instead of salt pork, ham hocks, smoked neck bones, or fatback.
- ▶ A diet rich in potassium may help to maintain healthy blood pressure. Eat potassium-rich beet greens, tomato products, soybeans, lima beans, winter squash, spinach, lentils, kidney beans, and split peas.
  - ▷ If you have problems with your kidneys you may need to restrict potassium. Talk to your health care provider to determine how much potassium is right for you.

Fruit Group

Any fruit or 100-percent fruit juice counts as part of the fruit group. You can eat fruit fresh, canned, frozen, or dried. Cut them up, eat them whole or puree them into a smoothie.

- ▶ Eat fruits raw, as juice with no sugar added, or canned in their own juice. Avoid canned fruit in heavy syrup.
- ▶ Eat pieces of fruit, rather than drinking fruit juice. Pieces of fruit are more filling.
- ▶ Buy fruit juice that is 100-percent juice, with no added sugar.
- ▶ To increase fiber intake, choose whole or cut-up fruits more often as snacks or with meals, instead of juice.
- ▶ Prune juice, bananas, cantaloupe, honeydew, prunes, dried peaches or apricots, orange juice, and plantains are all rich in potassium which may help to maintain healthy blood pressure.

Milk Group

All fluid milk products and many foods made from milk are considered part of this food group. Regardless of the fat content all types of milk have the same amount of carbohydrate—except cheese. It has none. Nutritionally, cheese is closer to meat, so you can find cheese in the fish, poultry, and meat group.

- ▶ Choose fat-free (skim) or low-fat (1 percent) milk, yogurt, and cheese.
- ▶ Eat low-fat or fat-free yogurt, and choose calcium-fortified frozen yogurt or ice milk.

▶ If you don't like the taste of milk, choose other calcium sources such as calcium-fortified foods and beverages, such as fortified breakfast cereals and juice, sardines, or tofu made with calcium. But move the food into the appropriate food group. For example, calcium fortified orange juice goes in the fruit group.

▶ If you can't drink milk because of lactose intolerance, eat hard cheese which doesn't have as much lactose. Or choose some of the lactose-free dairy products that are widely available.

◦━╫╾◦

What Is Lactose Intolerance?

Lactose intolerance occurs when you have a lower level of the enzyme lactase, which is needed to digest milk sugar.

Many African-Americans are avoiding dairy, particularly milk, because they think they are lactose intolerant. Usually, the notion of lactose intolerance and avoiding dairy comes from dietary habits learned early in life. As a result, Black folks are missing out on the many health benefits milk products offer. For example, there is a growing body of evidence that suggests dairy may play a role in reducing the risk of high blood pressure, heart disease, obesity, type 2 diabetes, and colon cancer. The National Medical Association, the nation's oldest and largest organization of African-American physicians, recommends that we consume 3-4 servings of low-fat dairy per day.

The good news is that lactose intolerance is not an all-or-nothing condition. It's a matter of degree. What we self diagnose as lactose intolerance is more closely related to lactose maldigestion—a condition that about 75 percent of all African-Americans have. But, by following a few simple strategies, you can take dairy foods daily and get all the health benefits without all the suffering.

Try these "Eight Great Tips For Tolerance" to help get your 3-4 recommended servings daily.

Eight Great Tips for Tolerance
1. **Start small.** Don't try to drink a glass of milk at one time. Begin with a small portion and slowly increase the serving size. For example, add a small amount of low fat milk to your coffee or hot chocolate.

2. **Spread it out.** Have small portions of dairy spread throughout the day. Add low-fat milk to your scrambled eggs or make grits with low-fat milk instead of water. Wrap beans and low-fat cheese in a tortilla for lunch; add a little shredded cheese to your salad.

3. **Pair the dairy.** Drink milk with meals instead of on an empty stomach. Solid foods slow digestion and allow your body more time to digest the lactose, which helps prevent symptoms.

4. **Say cheese.** When milk is made into cheese, most of the lactose is removed. Aged hard cheeses, such as cheddar, colby, Swiss and Parmesan, are particularly low in lactose. Add low-fat cheddar to your favorite cornbread recipe or serve rice and beans with colby.

5. **Get a little culture.** Cultured dairy products, such as yogurt with live active cultures, contain "friendly" bacteria that help digest lactose. Incorporate non-fat yogurt into a refreshing mango-and-banana smoothie for a great-tasting way to start the day

6. **Reduce it.** Look for lactose-free or lactose-reduced milk in the dairy case. It tastes the same as regular milk. Or "spike" your milk with a few lactase enzyme drops that are available in most drug stores. That will reduce the lactose in the milk.

7. **Make it easy.** Buy dairy digestive supplements (lactase caplets) at your drug store. If you take the caplets before you eat dairy foods, they can help you digest lactose easily.

8. **Go to the pros.** See your doctor for a diagnosis of your symptoms. Then, talk to your doctor or consult with a registered dietitian to learn how you can incorporate dairy foods into your diet.

Fish, Poultry, and Meat Group

Meat, poultry, and fish—and anything made from them—are part of this group. Eggs fit here, too. And because cheese is nutritionally closer to meat than to milk, it can be found in this group, as well. Choose fat-free or low-fat cheese, and lean meat and poultry cuts. But, if you're concerned about cholesterol—and you should be—limit even low-fat versions of these foods in favor of fish. It contains healthier oils. Also watch the sodium content of foods in this group. You're probably aware that processed meats such as ham, sausage, frankfurters, and luncheon or deli meats, have added sodium. But you may not realize that fresh chicken, turkey, and pork are often enhanced with a solution containing salt, so they may have added sodium as well. Check the label for statements like "self-basting," which means that sodium solution has been added to the product.

Getting enough protein is important, and eating foods from this group is one way to do so. But dietary guidelines suggest that you eat no more than 7 ounces from the meat group each day. When you make your daily meal plan, include a total of 5 to 7 ounces of fish, eggs, cheese or meat.

▶ Buy cuts of beef, pork, ham, and lamb that have only a little fat on them. Look for the words "loin" or "round" in their names.

▶ Buy ground beef that is at least 90 percent lean.

▶ Cook and eat chicken or turkey without the skin.

▶ Trim most of the visible fat from meat before cooking and trim the remaining fat before eating.

▶ Eat no more than three egg yolks per week—the yolk contains all the cholesterol in the egg.

▶ One serving of meat should weigh between 2 and 3 ounces after cooking.

Fats Group

Oils, solid fats, and soft margarine are part of the fat group, as you would expect. But this category also includes things like mayonnaise and certain salad dressings, as well as nuts and avocados, which have a high oil content, too. Most liquid oils are high in monounsaturated or polyunsaturated fats and low in saturated fats. Coconut oil, palm oil, and palm kernel oil are the exceptions; they're high in saturated fats. All oils from plant sources (vegetable and nut oils) are cholesterol free. But unless the food is high in omega-3 fatty acids, use it sparingly. Make 3 to 5 servings a day your limit. A serving is about a teaspoon of oil or a tablespoon of salad dressing. If you're eating very oily food, use less added fat in other foods. For example, a slice of bacon is the equivalent of a teaspoon of oil.

▶ Make most of your fat sources from healthy fats, such as those found in nuts, avocados, and olive and canola oils.

▶ Limit bacon grease and solid fats like butter, stick margarine, shortening, and lard, as well as foods that contain these fats.

▶ Check the Nutrition Facts Label to keep saturated fats and trans fats low.

▶ Remember, all types of fat are high in calories so limit them to small amounts.

How Much Is a Serving

Food Group	Samples of Serving Sizes
Milk	1 cup milk or buttermilk 1/2 frozen yogurt or evaporated milk 3/4 cup fortified soy milk 1 cup yogurt, plain or made with low-calorie sweetener
Fruit	1 medium peach, apple, or orange 1 1/2 cup watermelon 17 muscadines or 15 grapes 1/2 cup orange or grapefruit juice 1/2 cup fruit juice
Vegetable	1 1/2 cup cooked vegetables (carrots, green beans, etc.) 3 cups salad or raw vegetables 1 cup vegetable juice 1 1/2 cups cooked kale, poke salad, collard greens, or turnips.
Starch	1 slice of bread 1/2 cup corn, peas, lima beans, black-eyed peas, or succotash 1/3 cup rice, pasta, potato, or other cooked grains 1/2 cup dry cereal 1/2 cup grits 1 biscuit (2 □″ across) 1 piece cornbread (2″ square) 1/3 cup yam, sweet potato
Fish, poultry, meat, cheese	1 oz catfish, whiting, porgies or salmon 1 oz turkey or chicken 1 oz beef, goat, lamb or pork 1 oz cheddar cheese 1/4 cup cottage cheese
Fats	1 teaspoon oil, margarine, butter 1 tablespoons salad dressing 10 peanuts 2 tablespoons avocado 1 slice bacon
Sweets	1/2 cup ice cream 1 slice plain cake (2″ square) 5 vanilla wafers 1/2 cup pudding 1 tablespoon regular jam or jelly

Sweets and Desserts

Small amounts of sweets can be included in a healthy diet—even if you have diabetes—so feel free to have a small dessert at the end of a healthy meal. But be aware that most of the calories in cakes, pies, and cookies come from carbohydrates and fat, often unhealthy saturated fat and trans fat. Check labels and recipes and choose options that contain healthy carbs and fat.

A sugar trap to avoid is sweet drinks. Regular soda, sweetened fruit drinks, sweet tea, Kool-Aid, and sports drinks are all high in sugar. You can try drinks made with sugar substitutes, but they have zero nutritive value. Drink water instead and get the added benefit of beautifully hydrated skin, glossy hair, and healthy kidneys.

▶ Keep the amount of sweets and desserts within your carbohydrate allowance by substituting sweets and desserts for starch, fruit, or milk in your diet.

▶ Use caution when choosing low-fat or fat-free desserts; they often have more total carbohydrates.

▶ Control portions sizes. Enjoy a thin slice of cake instead of a 3-inch hunk.

▶ Limit sweets and desserts to one serving per day.

▶ Remember desserts made with honey and syrup affect your blood glucose the same way sugar does.

▶ Replace regular sugar with a sugar substitute such as stevia, Splenda, or Equal.

▶ Use sugar-free powdered mixes for Kool-Aid, lemonade, punch, and other fruit flavored drinks.

Your Personal Diabetes Soul Food Pyramid

You can create your own diabetes pyramid that includes the kinds of foods you enjoy—soul food, Caribbean food, health food, raw food, whatever you like. Doing it yourself means you never have to feel deprived of your favorite dishes (though you may have to modify your recipe or your portions). The more you enjoy what you eat, the less restricted you'll feel.

1. Determine how many carbohydrate choices you can have per meal. To do this, look at the chart on page 84 and find your situation. This will tell you the number of carbohydrate choices you have for each food group.

Carbohydrate Choices Per Day Divided by Food Group

Women	To lose weight	To control weight	For active individuals
Milk	1 – 2	2	2 – 3
Fruit	2	2 – 3	3
Vegetables	1 – 2	2	2
Starch	4 – 6	6 – 8	8 – 10
Men	To lose weight	To control weight	For active individuals
Milk	2	2 – 3	3
Fruit	2 – 3	3	3
Vegetables	2	2	3
Starch	6 – 8	8 – 10	10 – 12

Modified from American Diabetic Association

2. Now write in the number of servings you can have in the correct box in the pyramid. (A blank sample is found at the end of this chapter.) If you are a female who needs to lose weight, your pyramid will look like this:

Sample Diabetes Pyramid

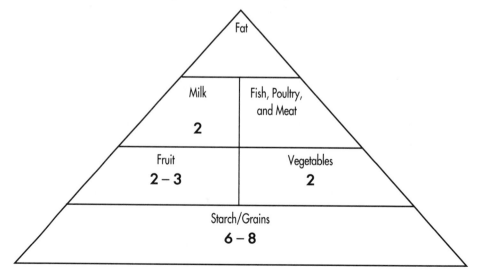

3. Note the foods you eat most often. In what area of the pyramid do your favorites fit? Remember that cheese counts as a meat, and starchy vegetables like peas, corn, and sweet potatoes go in the grain group.

4. Now use the meal planning chart at the end of this chapter to plan your menu for each day. Spread out your choices so that you're eating at least three meals at day. You can add up to three snacks as well. Try to get some protein at each meal and snack. Refer to the serving size chart to determine your portions.

When you're done, your diabetes soul-food menu for a given day might look like the one on page 86. Notice that there's a place on it to note your blood-sugar reading. You will need to check your blood sugars two hours after eating to make sure that your blood sugar stays under control. According to the American Diabetes Association, it should be less than 180 mg/dl two hours after eating. If it's higher, adjust your food choices.

It won't take long to get the hang of creating a meal plan this way—especially as you get more familiar with serving sizes for the foods you enjoy. Study the lists at the back of this book and highlight your favorites. If you want to explore other options, check out the next chapter to learn the carb counting method and glycemic index option. Try all three and select the meal planning process that works best for your lifestyle.

Power Points

☞ The Diabetes Food Guide Pyramid is one of three very successful meal planning strategies.

☞ In the Diabetes Food Pyramid, all foods containing carbohydrate are proportioned to provide 15 grams of carbohydrate.

☞ The Diabetes Soul-Food Pyramid was designed to incorporate ethnic foods that don't often show up on diabetes food lists—but are acceptable options for diabetes patients.

☞ The National Medical Association recommends African-Americans consume 3-4 servings of low-fat dairy per day. Research suggests that dairy may play a role in reducing the risk of high blood pressure, heart disease, obesity, type 2 diabetes, and colon cancer.

Sample Diabetes Soul Food Menu			
My Day	**Date**: 10/1		
Meal	Diabetes Soul Food Pyramid Choices:	Food and Serving:	SMBG: Time after meal: reading
Breakfast	1/2 milk choice 1/2 milk choice 1 fruit choice 1 grain choice 1 meat serving	Café au lait made with 1/2 cup milk and 1/2 cup coffee and 1 splenda 1/2 vanilla yogurt, non-fat with lo-cal sweetner mixed with 1/2 cup chopped raw mango 1/2 cup yellow grits served with 1 ounce sharp cheddar cheese	2 hours: 120
Snack	No snack		
Lunch	1 fruit choice 1 vegetable choice 1 1/2 grain choice 1 meat serving 1/2 grain choice	1 peach 1 1/2 cup cooked okra added to 1 cup chili con carne/beans, canned served with: 1/4 inch slice of French bread	
Snack	1 milk choice 1 grain choice 1 meat serving	1 cup buttermilk 5 Triscuits with: 1 ounce low-fat Colby cheese	
Dinner	1 vegetable choice 1 meat serving 2 grain choices 1/2 grain choice	1 1/2 cups McKenzie's pole beans, cut 4 ounces chicken (no skin) with 2 Dumplings (2 inch x 2 inch) and 1/4 cup brown gravy mix	

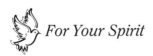 *For Your Spirit*

Your Daily Bread

Keep falsehood and lies far from me;
Give me neither poverty nor riches,
But give me only my daily bread.

—Proverbs 30:8

The foundation for a healthy life includes a few simple things—air, water, food, shelter, and clothing. With the exception of a growing number of homeless folks, most Americans are so accustomed to having the basics that we take it for granted that we have a bed to sleep in or that the fridge has something in it that we can eat. For most of us, it's not that we don't have enough for our basic survival. It's that we have so much.

Nowhere is that more evident than when we eat out. The stack of pancakes we order is the size of a small cake. We're offered quarts of soda to drink with our half-pound cheeseburgers. The coffee comes with three inches of whipped cream on top. Super-size is now the norm. And its showing in our super-size clothes and super-size health problems.

The proverb above is an apt one to remember when you order a meal. It is, frankly, a falsehood that an extra large drink and order of fries is truly an "extra value." Yes, you spend relatively less money, but it has a health cost that can't be calculated. And you can't afford to lie to yourself that "you won't eat it all" if you know you'll reheat the rest of it in the microwave later.

We have to maintain the same mindfulness at home, as well. We say grace before meals because we are grateful to have food to eat—rightly so when so many folks are hungry. But when we lift our heads from prayer and look at a table that's nearly buckling under the weight of the platters, we have to think twice about what is enough.

Truly, the key to good health and nutrition is "neither poverty nor riches." Be thankful that you have food to eat, but don't overdo it. A healthful diet means eating enough good food to give you the energy you need to get you through the day. That's your daily bread.

Your "daily bread" does not have to be dry and boring. In fact it *should* be delicious—every dish prepared with care, attention, and love, and every bite savored and enjoyed. Why bother to cook or eat food that is tasteless and boring? You won't even remember you ate it, much less feel very thankful for having it. It's an affront to God's blessing.

A diabetes patient today can be grateful that the disease can be controlled with a diet that isn't restrictive and can include good food—even sweet delights. Even if you are trying to lose weight, it's possible to eat well and feel satisfied. When you eat food you love—preferably with the people you love—you'll realize that "enough" really is enough.

Food Pyramid

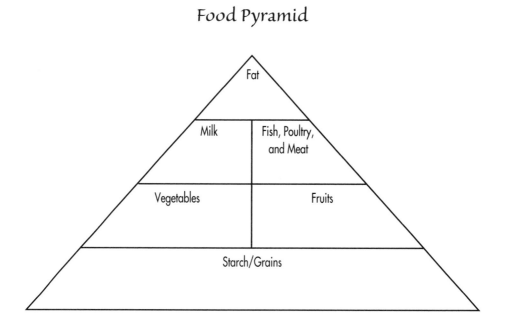

Use your pyramid to plan your meals. Make copies of this chart and use it daily.

Diabetes Soul Food Menu

My Day	Date:		
Meal	Diabetes Soul Food Pyramid Choices:	Food and Serving:	SMBG: Time after meal: reading
Breakfast			
Snack			
Lunch			
Snack			
Dinner			

7 OTHER MEAL PLANNING STRATEGIES

When the ADA announced that there was no longer one "right" way for a diabetes patient to eat, it created a way for people to individualize their diets so they could eat what felt right to them and still maintain proper blood-sugar control. While the diabetes pyramid has been a familiar old standby, there are two other excellent methods of meal planning that many people find effective.

Carbohydrate Counting

Carbohydrate counting gained popularity as a meal planning method after the Diabetes Control and Complications Trial (DCCT) reported that carbohydrate counting was the most successful meal-planning method used by the study participants. The study, conducted by the National Institute of Diabetes and Digestive and Kidney Diseases (NIDDK), showed that keeping blood glucose levels as close to normal as possible slows the onset and progression of eye, kidney, and nerve diseases caused by diabetes.

Because carbohydrate counting is not a diet but a meal planning tool, it gives you greater flexibility in your meal choices and helps you to understand how food affects your blood glucose level. Now let's look at carbohydrate counting in more detail.

Everything that you eat, with the exception of pure animal protein and fat, has some carbohydrate content. Remember that when you eat foods containing carbohydrates, like corn bread, grits, peaches, milk, or even collard greens, your body breaks these foods down into sugar—glucose. The glucose then enters into your bloodstream, where it can be used to energize the cells of the body. The more carbohydrate-containing foods you eat at a meal, the more glucose will enter the bloodstream.

Also remember that in type 2 diabetes, your body doesn't produce enough insulin to take the glucose out of the bloodstream and allow it to be used for energy. Or your body does make enough insulin, but the insulin is unable to do its job properly (insulin resistance). It's often said that a picture is worth a thousand words, so to better understand what's going on in your body and why you need to change the way you eat, picture a clogged drain.

We've all experienced a clogged drain at one time or another. If the clog isn't too bad and the water is running slowly, the sink will drain. It may not even be obvious that the drain is clogged. But turn the faucet on high and fill the sink up, and it will take a very long time for that water to go down. Or in the worst-case scenario, it won't move at all.

This is basically what happens in your body as a result of insulin resistance. If you eat small amounts of foods containing carbohydrates at a meal (like the drips of water in the clogged drain), your body will work more efficiently. Your blood glucose levels will not go up as high. On the other hand, if you chow down on corn bread, potato salad, macaroni and cheese, and sweet potatoes all in one meal—well, that's like turning the faucet on high. Your glucose levels will spike and take a long time to return to normal. To make matters worse, before there is a significant drop in your glucose levels, you get hungry and eat again. The result? Your glucose levels rises even higher.

Now don't misunderstand: this does not mean you can never ever indulge in a piece of warm, made-from-scratch, mouth-watering corn bread. But you certainly must monitor your portions and consider the carbohydrate content. Experts tell us that it is the total amount of carbohydrates eaten at a meal, and not the source or type, that impacts glucose control. So whether you choose to count each gram of carbohydrate in your food or use the "choice method" of carbohydrate counting, you will learn to include a variety of your favorite foods and maintain good glucose control.

The Choice Method of Carbohydrate Counting

The Diabetes Soul Food Pyramid is a great place to start when using the choice method for counting carbohydrates. Take a look at the Diabetes Soul Food Pyramid on page 76. A carbohydrate choice is a serving of food from the starch, fruit, vegetable, or milk group. Each serving counts as one carbohydrate choice and gives you 15 grams of carbs.

It's reasonable for most adults to consume 3–4 carbohydrate choices at each meal and eat 1 to 2 carb choices for snacks. Look at the following table to determine your best choices. To ensure you get enough food from each food group, the chart suggests how many carbohydrate servings you should have from each food group every day. Don't forget to complete your meal by adding 2 to 3 ounces of fish, poultry, meat, or meat substitute.

To further determine your best choices, check your blood glucose levels two hours after eating a meal. According to the American Diabetes Association a blood glucose level less than 180 mg/dl is an indicator of good diabetes control. If you are not achieving your goals, see a registered dietitian or certified diabetes educator, who will help you find your best choices.

Carbohydrate Choices Per Day Divided by Food Group

Women	To lose weight	To control weight	For active individuals
Milk	1 – 2	2	2 – 3
Fruit	2	2 – 3	3
Vegetables	1 – 2	2	2
Starch	4 – 6	6 – 8	8 – 10
Men	To lose weight	To control weight	For active individuals
Milk	2	2 – 3	3
Fruit	2 – 3	3	3
Vegetables	2	2	3
Starch	6 – 8	8 – 10	10 – 12

Modified from American Diabetic Association

To determine what a serving size is, you'll need to measure your food. I know that sounds like a lot of work, but as in every aspect of life, you get what you pay for. The payoff in this case will be good blood glucose control. Usually, once you measure your food for a while and start to get a feel for what 1/3 cup of rice or a cup of greens looks like, measuring will be less necessary. (Just don't let those portion sizes creep up.)

If you still can't fathom the idea of measuring your food, then at least aim for what I call "repeatability." In other words, always use the same cups, dishes, utensils, and so on, for the same foods. If you fill your favorite Tupperware bowl with cereal every morning, and your blood glucose levels two hours after breakfast are continually higher than your target, try filling that same favorite Tupperware bowl half full. Just remember, the most accurate method of controlling portions is to use measuring cups

Converting Carb Grams to Carb Choices	
Carbohydrate Grams	Carbohydrate Choices
0–5	0
6–10	1/2
11–20	1
21–25	1 1/2
26–35	2
36–40	2 1/2
41–50	3
51–55	3 1/2
56–65	4
66–70	4 1/2
71–80	5
Source: American Diabetes Association	

and spoons. When you measure your food at home, it also makes it easier to choose correct portions when away from home.

There will be times when you are eating foods that contain more or less than 15 grams of carbohydrates. The following chart will show you how to convert these foods into carbohydrate choices. Remember, 15 grams of carb equals 1 carbohydrate choice.

The Gram Method of Carbohydrate Counting

Counting carbohydrates by grams is a more precise method of controlling your carbohydrate intake than the choice method. This method gives you greater flexibility, especially when you're eating prepackaged foods. See the following table to determine your suggested carbohydrate gram intake.

Carbohydrate Grams Per Meal			
	To Lose Weight	To Control Weight	For Active Individuals
Women	45–60	60–75	75–90
Men	60–75	75–90	90–105
If you eat snacks between meals, subtract carbohydrate grams from a meal.			
Source: American Diabetes Association			

To truly master carbohydrate counting, you will need to learn how to read the nutrition facts panel found on food labels.

The nutrition facts information shows you what a serving size is and how many grams of carbohydrates that serving will give you. The nutrition facts panel has a great deal of information on it but for now, we will examine only the information that will help with carbohydrate counting.

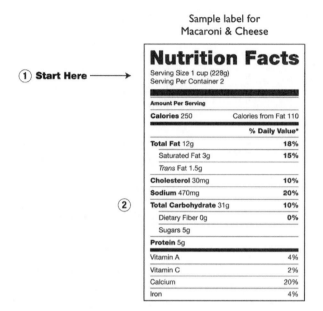

Sample label for
Macaroni & Cheese

Look at the sample label for macaroni and cheese. (For the purpose of illustration, this is a simplified label.) Starting at the top, look at the serving size is 1 cup; there are two servings per container. Next, the "Amount Per Serving" will tell you the amount of calories and nutrients in a single serving. At number 2, you will notice that the total carbohydrates (found in bold print) is 31 grams. One cup of macaroni and cheese has 31 grams of carbohydrate. In lighter print directly under "Total Carbohydrate," you will notice Dietary Fiber and Sugar. The fiber and sugar grams are included in the total grams of carbohydrate. If a food item contains sugar alcohol, it will be listed here also. Remember, it is the total amount of carbohydrates that impacts your glucose levels. Now, if you've been told "just stay away from sugar," think about that advice. If you only focus on the sugar content in the mac and cheese, you'll think you're getting 5 grams—not bad. But unless you count total carbs, there will be 26 grams of carbohydrates you didn't count. And that 26 grams of carbohydrate will make your glucose level rise higher than anticipated. Get the idea? Controlling total carbohydrates is the key to successfully controlling diabetes.

The Glycemic Index

In conversations about blood-sugar control, one can't help but discuss the glycemic index (GI) which was developed in the 1980s by David J.A. Jenkins, MD, PhD, an expert on dietary fiber.

GI is a measurement of how fast a particular carbohydrate raises blood sugar as compared to a standard amount of glucose. A standard amount of glucose will raise blood sugar faster than any other food, and is rated as 100. All other foods are rated from 0 to 100 depending on how the food compares to the glucose standard. Foods with a high GI will raise your blood sugar quickly, while a low GI food, which is absorbed more slowly, will raise your blood sugar more slowly.

Unfortunately, GI is more complicated than it might seem. Even foods with the same carbohydrate content can affect your blood sugar differently, depending on the GI of the food. And a food may have a different GI depending on how it's prepared—so you count the GI of a potato differently if you boil it than if you bake it. It's a lot to keep track of.

However, there is a growing body of research that indicates that the GI may provide an additional benefit in the management of diabetes. Let's look at the pros and cons to using the GI.

Glycemic Index of Selected Foods

Food	Glycemic Index	Food	Glycemic Index
Biscuits	92	Pigeon peas	22
Black-eyed peas	33	Plantain	40
Butter beans	28	Potato, Mashed	67
Cabbage	32	Potato, Russet, baked	94
Collard greens	32	Potato, Sweet	48
Cornbread	75.5	Rice, Arborio	69
Grits	69	Rice, Basmati	58
Kale	32	Rice, Brown	66
Lima beans	32	Rice, Jasmine	109
Mango	60	Rice, Long grain	56
Mustard greens	32	Rice, Long grain parboiled	68
Okra	32	Rice, White	69
Papaya	60	Turnip	72

The Benefits

A low-GI diet seems to lead to lower fasting blood-sugar levels. It also reduces hemoglobin A1c, which suggests that blood-sugar control is maintained over a longer period of time. There is also some evidence that a low-GI diet may lead to less hunger, which can prevent overeating and weight gain. Other possible benefits of a low-GI diet include lower insulin levels, heightened mental alertness, and enhanced sports performance.

The Problems

GI is not a precise or absolute measurement. Similar foods from different manufacturers will vary in their GI number, sometimes by as much as 20 percent. Many factors appear to affect the GI of a food. These factors include processing, preparation, variety, origin, and ripeness of a food.

Processing foods by grinding, rolling, pressing, or mashing can increase a food's GI—thus baked potatoes have a lower GI than mashed potatoes, for example. Basmati rice, long-grain white rice, brown rice, and arborio rice have different GIs. Foods from different parts of the world will have different GIs: potatoes produced in Idaho will have a different GI than potatoes produced in Ireland. Ripeness of a fruit or vegetable will also affect a food's GI. For example, green bananas have a lower GI than ripe bananas. Stranger still, cooling a food can cause the reduction in the food's GI. Letting a baked potato cool after cooking it lowers its GI.

Additionally, everyone's blood sugar reacts differently to different GI foods. For example, sweet potato is considered a low GI food but how your blood sugar reacts to it might be different than how someone else's blood sugar reacts. The best way to learn how a food reacts with you is to check your blood sugar two hours after your meal and develop your personal list of low GI foods.

The GI is also a relative measurement. The GI of a food depends on the standard that it is compared to. Many times a standard glucose dose is used which has a GI of 100. Compared to a glucose dose, white bread has a GI of 70. But sometimes white bread is used as the standard reference, which means it has a GI of 100. This means that all the foods tested against white bread will have a GI that is 40 percent higher than they would have using the glucose standard.

Many researchers are concerned that people may think that foods with a low GI are healthier than foods with a high GI, and choose foods based only on the GI. For example, carrots have high GI but have tremendous health benefits. Another worrisome example is that French fries have a lower GI than plain baked potatoes, when obviously the baked potato is healthier for you than a fried one.

Another problem with teaching GI to the average patient is that, as you can see, it's complicated—much more so than the exchange method of meal planning or carbohydrate counting. That doesn't mean it isn't doable. It just takes effort—and you may find that the effort pays off handsomely for you. If you plan to use the glycemic index method, keep in mind the following:

▶ Do not forget to look at the total nutrition of a food. Just because it is high GI does not mean it does not have other nutritional benefits, or just because it is a low GI does not mean that it is necessarily healthy.

▶ If you choose a high GI food, combine it with a protein or fat to lower the GI. For example, have a baked potato topped with low-fat chili.

▶ Eat whole grains, because they tend to have a lower GI due to their fiber content.

▶ Eat lots of fresh fruits and vegetables, most of which are low GI foods.

▶ If quick meals are important to you, choose parboiled rice instead of instant rice, because instant rice has a higher GI than parboiled.

▶ Eating cooled potatoes in foods such as potato salad lowers the GI. However, watch the mayo or dressing you use to prepare the salad.

▶ Instead of creamy dressings consider those with vinegar; they will slow digestion as much as a high-fat dressing but without the added calories. Slowing digestion will lower the GI.

▶ Portion size is just as important as GI because the more you eat, the higher your blood sugar will go regardless of the GI of the foods you are eating.

▶ Check your blood sugars two hours after a meal to find out how your body deals with a food or meal.

The Plate Method

If all of these meal planning methods seem confusing try the plate method. There's no addition, subtraction, calculating percentages, or weighing involved. You're not really counting anything. It's just you, your food, and your plate.

It works like this: When you get ready to serve yourself a meal, make sure half the plate is full of non-starchy vegetables. A quarter of the plate is for your starchy vegetable; the other quarter is for fish, poultry or meat. That's it.

It's not as exact as the other method, but it's a good start toward helping you control portions. Filling half the plate with non-starches automatically reduces your carb count. And if you keep it to that one plate per meal, it will reduce your calorie count, too. (Note this is called the *plate* method, not the *platter* method. If you want to keep your portions under control, don't use the biggest plate you can find. It may help to buy some of the paper plates that are sectioned, and use those until you get used to what your new portions look like.)

It may be the method you want to use until you get the hang of one of the others. And certainly if you aren't able to control your diabetes this way, you'll need to try one of the other methods that's more precise. But this method alone can make a difference. And any change is better than no change at all.

Power Points

🕊 Carbohydrate counting gives you greater flexibility in meal choices.

🕊 Experts agree that it is the total amount of carbohydrate eaten at a meal, not the source or type that impacts glucose control.

🕊 The most accurate method of controlling portions is to use measuring cups and spoons.

🕊 The glycemic index (GI) may provide an additional benefit in the management of diabetes.

🕊 High GI foods raise blood sugar quickly, while low GI foods are absorbed more slowly and raise blood sugar more slowly.

🕊 Low GI foods are not necessarily healthier than high GI foods.

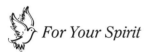 *For Your Spirit*

More Than One Way to Get a Job Done

The story of Jesus and the miracle of the loaves and fishes is a lesson in faith as well as spiritual ingenuity.

You know the story. As Jesus and the disciples traveled, ministering and performing works of wonder, people began to follow him wherever he went, waiting for a miracle. One day, up on a mountain, Jesus looked down to find some 5,000 people waiting below. Waiting for him to...do something. Thirsting to hear or see something that fed their soul—with their bellies empty besides. First, he said, lets feed them.

He turned to his disciples and asked a trick question. Where could they buy enough to feed the hungry people. They couldn't imagine. They didn't have any money enough to feed all those mouths. There was a boy in the crowd who'd thought to bring a lunch—two fish and five little loaves of bread—but even if he shared, it wouldn't feed those multitudes. Or would it? Jesus' question wasn't really about buying anything. It was a test of the extent of the people's faith.

He took the bread and fish and began to pray, giving thanks for it. Then He had the disciples start passing out food—and keep passing out food until everyone was fed. The people kept coming, the food kept coming until everyone was full and still there was more. Everyone marveled, including the disciples.

The whole point of this miracle was to show the power of faith. But it also demonstrated that there is more than one way to do a thing. In this case, there was the traditional way to feed a crowd—go to the market, buy up lots of food, and fire up the stove. And then there was the spiritual way: take what you have on hand, bless it, and do the best you can with it.

God gives us choices and opportunities—every chance in the world to do the right thing. Often there is more than one path to what is "right"—so even if we make a wrong turn, by the Grace of God, we can often find our way around to where we need to be. This is as true when it comes to taking care of our physical bodies as it is for our spiritual bodies.

When we stray from the path or fall off the wagon, it's easy to give up. "Oh forget it," we say after another week of standing on a scale that won't seem to budge. "This diet isn't working." When we give up, though, we aren't exercising either our faith in God or our confidence in our god-given ability to "make a way out of no way"—both of which have been tested and proven over generations.

Instead of losing faith, we have to remember that there's always more than one way to get a job done. If the diabetes pyramid doesn't work for you, maybe you need to try carb counting. If walking doesn't help you feel healthier, maybe a yoga class will. If God wants us to do something, he'll make a way for it to get done. We just have to open our eyes and see the possibilities we've been blessed with.

Exercising our faith and truly believing that God will help us find a way to heal is the first step—and the second and the last. When it comes to taking care of any of our needs—for physical sustenance, for health, for spiritual growth—we must remember to keep looking for the right way to do it.

8 WHAT'S IN A NAME?
FOOD LABELS DEMYSTIFIED

In the previous chapters you learned all about meal planning strategies that will help you successfully manage diabetes. You were even taught how to use the nutrition facts label for carbohydrate counting. But is that enough? Not really. In order to truly be successful at managing your food intake you must be able to understand all the information found on the nutrition facts label.

If you've attempted to read the nutrition facts label in the past and failed to understand the information, then you're not alone. How many grams of fat or sodium are considered high? What does the percent daily value (%DV) mean? I don't eat 2000 calories a day so how can I use the percent daily value? And what does low-fat mean anyway? The labels on your food hold the answers to all of these questions and more. They'll be revealed as we demystify the food label.

Nutrition Facts Label Work Sheet

Let's check out a nutrition label. It looks pretty complicated, with all the facts and figures, but it's actually pretty harmless once you get to know it. Once you walk through it step by step, you will be able to use the information more easily and effectively—and tell at a glance what's going on with what's going into your body.

The first place to start when you look at the nutrition label is the serving size and number of servings in the package. Serving sizes are based on the amount typically eaten. However, that is not to say that what you consider a serving is the same as a typical serving. Pay attention to the serving size, including how many servings there are in the food package, and compare it to how much *you* actually eat. In the sample label, a serving is one cup. If you ate the whole package, you would eat two cups. That doubles the calories and other nutrient numbers, including the %DV.

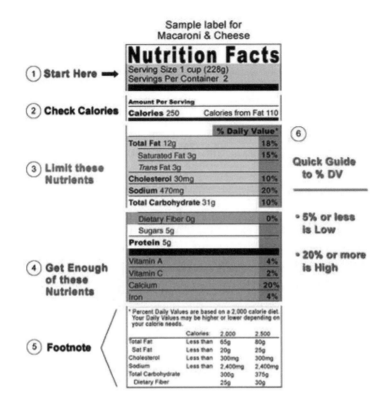

Sample label for Macaroni & Cheese

The calorie information tells you the number of calories in a single serving and how many calories come from fat. In our sample label there are 250 calories per serving and 110 calories from fat. That means that about half of the calories come from fat. If you ate the whole package, you would eat 500 calories—220 calories would come from fat.

Fat, cholesterol, and sodium should be limited in the diet if you want to avoid heart disease, some cancers, or high blood pressure. To keep your intake as low as possible, be sure the "% Daily Value" of these nutrients is less than 5%. (Another easy way to keep your fat intake low is to aim for no more than 3 grams of total fat per 100 calories.)

You should try to get enough essential nutrients such as calcium, iron, and vitamins A and C, as well as other components such as dietary fiber. Try to average 100% for each one of these nutrients each day. A food item with 20% or more of these essential nutrients is high in those nutrients. In the sample, the daily value for calcium is 20%, which means the macaroni and cheese is high in calcium.

The footnote is only found on larger packages and provides general dietary information about important nutrients. When the full footnote does appear, it will always be the same. It doesn't change from product to product.

The quick guide to %DV can help you evaluate your daily food intake and determine if a serving of food is high or low in a nutrient. You do not need to know how to calculate percentages. The label does the math for you—5% DV or less is low and 20% DV or more is high.

Finding Hidden Sugars

Have you ever wondered why there are carbs in meat like frankfurters, bologna, or other processed meats? Or why your blood glucose levels go up higher than usual after eating these foods? Hidden sugar is most likely the cause. Often times, food manufactures list these ingredients using unfamiliar terms, but with a little detective work you can find hidden carbs in your food. Here is a list of the different names you might find in an ingredient list—all of which mean "sugar."

Amasake or amazake	Honey
Barley malt syrup	Invert sugar
Brown rice syrup	Lactose
Brown sugar	Levulose
Carob powder	Maltose
Confectioner's sugar	Malt syrup
Corn sweetener	Maple syrup
Corn syrup	Molasses
Date sugar	Raw sugar
Dextrose	Rapadura
Evaporated whole cane juice	Refined sugar
Fructose	Sucanat
Fruit juice concentrates	Sucrose
Galactose	Sugar
Glucose	Syrup
High-fructose corn syrup	Turbinado sugar

You should also know how to find out if there are sugar alcohols in your food. They appear in the ingredient list as:

Erythritol   Malitol

Hydrogenated starch hydrolysates   Mannitol

Isomalt   Sorbitol

Lactitol   Xylitol

Many people believe they are "free food," because sugar-free gums and candy include them. These reduced-calorie sweeteners aren't exactly carbohydrate free, however, so they can still cause your blood glucose levels to go up. Sugar alcohols actually provide about half the calories of other carbohydrates because only about half of it is digested. This is particularly important because, if you are taking meal-time insulin and trying to fine tune your blood-glucose levels, you need to know the true number of carbs you are getting.

The following formula can help you determine how to count carbohydrates in food that contain sugar alcohols. You might want to get out your pencil for this—it requires a little math. First find the number of grams of sugar alcohols on the nutrition facts label and divide that number in half. Next, subtract that number from the total grams of carbohydrate, and then count the remaining grams.

Use this example from a meal-replacement bar:

Serving size: 1 bar

Total carbohydrate: 31g

Dietary fiber: 8g

Sugars: 0g

Sugar alcohol: 20g

There are 20 grams of sugar alcohol.

Divide that number in half.

$$20 \text{ g} \div 2 = 10\text{g}$$

There are 31 grams of total carbohydrate.

Subtract 10g from total carbohydrates.

$$31 \text{ g} - 10 \text{ g} = 21\text{g of total carbohydrate}$$
available to raise your
blood glucose levels

You only count 21g, which can be converted to 1 1/2 carbohydrate choices by using the table found on the Food Label Worksheet on page 100.

Keep in mind this tip only works if the Nutrition Facts Label provides you with the sugar alcohol information; sugar alcohols are voluntary information. If it's listed in the ingredients but not on nutrition label, you won't be able to use this formula. You just have to count total carbs.

Sugar is not the only ingredient that is often found disguised by an unfamiliar name. Trans fat is also sometimes hidden. If you eat only trans fat-free foods you aren't consuming any trans fat at all, right? Wrong. The law states that a food containing half a gram (0.5 g) or less of trans fat can be listed as zero grams on the label and the manufacturer can call it "trans fat free." But that half gram of trans fat is in there and these small amounts can add up throughout the day. How do you know if you're eating trans fats? Look at the ingredient list for hydrogenated oils or partially hydrogenated oils.

For those on meal-time insulin, fiber offers another opportunity to adjust your total carbohydrate intake. Because the body can't digest fiber, you can subtract half of the fiber grams from the total carbohydrate amount. Don't bother unless the food has more than 5 grams of fiber. If you look at the same meal replacement bar from above, you'll see 8g of dietary fiber. Let's do the math.

There are 8 grams of fiber.

Divide that number in half

$$8 \text{ g} \div 2 = 4\text{g}$$

There are 31 grams of total carbohydrate.

Subtract 4g from total carbohydrates.

$$31\text{g} - 4\text{g} = 27\text{g of total carbohydrate}$$
available to raise your
blood glucose levels

Okay, I know what you're thinking: *What happens when there is fiber and sugar alcohol?* Well, then you simply subtract both. In this case you'd subtract 10g of sugar alcohol and 4g of fiber—14 grams from the 31 total grams of carbs.

Nutrition Claims

The Nutrition Labeling and Education Act of 1990 permits the use of label claims that characterize the level of a nutrient in a food. Nutrient claims describe the level of a substance in the product, using terms such as "free," "high," and "low." Or they compare the level of a nutrient in a food to that of another food, using terms such as "more," "reduced," and "lite." Sound confusing? Here are some tips that will help you make sense of it all.

FREE

Fat-free	less than 0.5 gram of fat per serving
Cholesterol-free	less than 2 milligrams of cholesterol per serving
Sodium-free	less than 5 milligrams of sodium per serving
Sugar-free	less than 0.5 grams of sugar per serving
Calorie-free	less than 5 calories per serving

Low

Low fat	3 grams of fat or less per serving
Low saturated fat	1 gram of saturated fat or less per serving
Low cholesterol	20 milligrams of cholesterol or less per serving
Low sodium	140 milligrams of sodium or less per serving
Low calorie	40 calories or less per serving

REDUCED OR LESS

Reduced/Less fat	at least 25% less fat than the regular food
Reduced/Less saturated fat	at least 25% less saturated fat than the regular food
Reduced/Less cholesterol	at least 25% less cholesterol than the regular food
Reduced or Less	at least 25% less sodium than the regular food
Reduced or Less sugar	at least 25% less sugar than the regular food
Reduced or Less calories	at least 25% fewer calories than the regular food
LIGHT OR LITE	1/3 fewer calories or 50% less fat than the regular food

Whole Grains

When the USDA updated the dietary guidelines and revamped the pyramid for Americans in 2005, they inadvertently started a new craze with manufacturers—the whole grain craze. The new guidelines say we should eat half of our grains—or at least 3 ounces a day—in the form of "whole grains." In response to these new changes, many food companies have started adding whole grains to their ingredient list—even in foods that are generally unhealthy. The snack food or cookie aisle tells the tale. You can find whole grain chips, crackers, and cookies boasting of their whole grain goodness. But don't be misled—these foods may still contain refined grains—and be loaded with sugar and fat to boot. Your best bet is to read the food label carefully, including the ingredient list, and make sure that whole wheat or another whole grain is the first ingredient. Ingredients are listed in order of weight, from most to least.

Food Safety and Handling

Along with all the required nutritional information, the FDA also requires food companies to tell consumers the best way to handle their products to prevent illness from bacterial growth and food-borne illnesses. Unpasteurized juice contains a warning that the product may contain harmful bacteria that "can cause serious illness in children, the elderly, and persons with weakened immune systems." After concerns with salmonella in certain populations, the FDA required that egg cartons put handling instructions on their labels that include "keep eggs refrigerated; cook eggs until yolks are firm; and cook foods containing eggs thoroughly." Meats and prepared foods often have handling instructions as well.

Another way that food safety is maintained is through product dating. A product package may have a "sell by" date which tells the store when to remove the product from the shelf. The "best if used by" date tells you when the quality of the product will start to decline; it's not necessarily an indication that the food is unsafe. The "use by" date is the only date that might make you think you shouldn't use the product. This one is usually found on perishable items such as meat, poultry, fish, eggs, and dairy products. Food dating is not required on any food except for infant formula and some baby food, so there is no uniform method of dating food.

As you can see, the Nutrition Facts Label and other information on food packaging provide you with a great deal of information that can impact your health. Understanding how to use the information on the label can empower you to better managing your diabetes and your overall health.

Power Points

☞ The Nutrition Facts Label can help you make healthful food choices.

☞ The %DV can help you evaluate if a serving of food is high or low in a particular nutrient.

☞ Fat, saturated fat, cholesterol, and sodium should be limited in the diet. To keep your intake as low as possible, make sure the %DV of these nutrients is less than 5%.

☞ You should try to get enough calcium, iron, and vitamins A and C, as well as fiber. Try to average 100%DV for each one of these nutrients each day. A food item with 20% or more of these nutrients is high in those nutrients.

☞ Sugar alcohols provide half the calories of other carbohydrates.

☞ Your body cannot digest fiber and therefore it does not make your blood glucose level rise.

☞ Read the ingredient list on the food label to find hidden sugar, saturated fat, and food allergens in the food. Ingredients are listed from most to least.

☞ Foods with health claims will also have limited amounts of fat, saturated fat, cholesterol, and sodium.

☞ Read the food label to determine how to properly store and prepare foods.

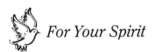 *For Your Spirit*

Second Chances

Alonzo Mourning's team, the Miami Heat, had defeated the Dallas Mavericks for the 2006 National Basketball Association championship, and the 6-foot-10-inch center had played a spectacular game that night. It was also his personal comeback as an NBA star after a brief career lapse due to health complications, so reporters clamored after him. He was the interview to get.

As his fans watched the interview, wanting to hear the star athlete's assessment of the basketball game, to their surprise, he spent most of the interview speaking about the importance of overcoming his illness—a life-threatening kidney disease that required him to have a transplant.

As he reflected on the days of pain and agony he endured while seeking to be cured, Mourning then recalled telling a close relative, "All the money and fame doesn't mean a thing without good health. I'd give up anything to get back my health. That's how important my health [is] to me."

He closed out his comments with an appreciation for another opportunity to enjoy a healthy and prosperous life. "I thank God that He has given me a second chance," he said.

If you think of it this way, a diagnosis of diabetes can be a second chance at life. If you haven't been paying attention to your diet, if you've been a little too sedentary, if you've been overdoing the sweets and underdoing the vegetables, finding out you have diabetes can be a wake-up call. If you're serious about being well, it can make you really—*really* this time—take the time to improve your eating habits, explore new cooking methods, take off a few extra pounds and develop an exercise routine.

In this way, diabetes is a blessing. Of course you may be able to think of some other blessings that you might rather receive, but having a second chance at life is an amazing, priceless gift.

9 ALTERNATE ROUTES: THE PROS AND CONS OF ALTERNATIVE TREATMENTS

In our grandparents' day, health was pretty simple: if you woke up in the morning "clothed in your right mind," you considered yourself well. Folks ate what they had, then worked it off in the factory or in the field. If you got "bad sick," you prayed—for a quick recovery or, if not that, an easy passing.

Today, staying healthy has become a full-time preoccupation for many of us. It's not just a matter of waking up in the morning and being grateful to move though the day. It's become a second job—watching every calorie and gram of fiber, exercising to meet exact weekly goals, chewing vitamins formulated especially for our age, gender, or health condition. As we get more conscious of our health, we also want to be more in control of it as well. We're not leaving it up to the doctor to take care of us. We're taking our health in our own hands.

This culture creates the perfect environment for the rise in alternative and complementary medicine. Sometimes these terms are used interchangeably, but alternative treatments include herbs, body work, specialized diets, and other treatments used for healthcare and healing *instead of* standard medical care; complementary care involves the use of alternative treatments *along with* standard medical care.

Back in the old days, alternative treatments—herbs, poultices, and other concoctions—were all we had. Once we gained better access to healthcare, our use of alternative treatments dropped. These days, however, studies show a steady increase in the use of alternative therapies among African-Americans. And there are a number of herbs, supplements, and diets that are being touted as ways to regulate or treat diabetes. Before you try any of them, you should know exactly what you are getting into.

The safest way to use unconventional therapies is as part of a comprehensive treatment plan that you develop with your doctor.

In fact, it is very important to talk with the folks on your diabetes dream team if you are taking or planning to use an alternative treatment. Unfortunately, African-Americans don't share this information with their doctors. In recent studies, only 40 percent of African-Americans (versus 55 percent of non-Hispanic whites) reported telling their doctors that they were using a complementary therapy. This can be a big problem, because some complementary therapies may interact poorly with your diabetes medication. Your diabetes dream team can make you aware of any potential interactions or side effects.

Let's look at some complementary diets and supplements that have been used in the treatment of diabetes. Starting with diets, we will review what the diet is, how it might help diabetes, and the evidence of the claims.

Diets

The Alkaline Diet

The diet is based on the fact that our body has a pH of 7.36 to 7.44, which makes it slightly alkaline. The idea is that your diet should also be slightly alkaline. People who recommend this diet say it can help you lose weight, increase your energy, and reduce your risk of heart disease and cancer.

The truth is that the body works very hard and very efficiently on its own to keep the blood at the proper pH—there's hardly need to alter your diet to try to affect the pH level. This diet does not include foods from all major food groups; it's not balanced. And there is no research-based evidence that shows the benefits of an alkaline diet. Eat a balanced diet but don't worry about balancing acids and bases; your body will do its job maintaining your pH.

The Food-Combining Diet

Food-combining theory says that different food groups are digested better when eaten in certain combinations. This diet promotes eating proteins and starches at separate meals. Vegetables can be eaten with both protein and starch, but fruits should be eaten alone. Its proponents say this diet will encourage weight loss and improved digestion of foods.

The truth is that there is no evidence that this diet is beneficial. In fact, it might be harmful. Because proteins and starches cannot be eaten together, one is often chosen over the other, which can cause a nutritional deficiency. For people with diabetes, this diet is the exact opposite of what is recommended for good blood-sugar control. Balancing a meal with both protein and carbohydrates means you'll end up consuming fewer carbs at that meal, resulting in more stable blood sugars and insulin levels. Don't worry about mixing proteins with carbohydrates; instead, enjoy that turkey on whole wheat.

The Macrobiotic Diet

This diet incorporates the Asian philosophy that foods are either yin (cooler) or yang (warmer) and that certain health conditions require food that will cool or warm you. The macrobiotic diet is vegetarian-based, consisting mainly of brown rice, whole grains, and vegetables. It has gained popularity among cancer patients who understand it to be an effective way to treat the disease. Currently, researchers are examining whether a macrobiotic diet can prevent or cure cancer, but no conclusive evidence has been found yet. Many people believe that macrobiotics can also prevent and treat diabetes and heart disease, but no research has been done.

Can a diet that is made up of mainly whole grains and vegetables be all that bad? The fact that it is very restrictive means it may cause deficiencies in some important nutrients such as protein, vitamin B12, iron, magnesium, and calcium.

The Raw Food Diet

Based on unprocessed and uncooked plant foods, the raw food diet consists of fresh fruits and vegetables, sprouts, seeds, nuts, grains, beans, dried fruit, and seaweed. Followers believe that heating a food above 116°F will destroy helpful enzymes in the food, but eating food raw or carefully dehydrated will increase energy, improve digestion, promote weight loss, and reduce your risk of chronic illnesses including diabetes.

It is naturally low in saturated and trans fats, which is good. But it still has some problems. First, this diet is very restrictive and could cause nutritional deficiencies of nutrients such as calcium, iron, B12, and protein. It takes a real commitment to make sure you are getting all the nutrients you need. There's the time commitment, too. No, you aren't cooking, but you will need to sprout your beans, grains, and seeds; dehydrate your foods; soak your nuts and dried fruit; juice your fruits and vegetables; and find the the ingredients that are needed (for example young coconut milk or date sugar).

The enzymes needed for digestion don't come from your foods; they come from your digestive tract, so it doesn't really matter whether or not the enzymes in our food is destroyed during cooking. In fact, some nutrients, such as beta-carotene found in carrots, are more available in cooked foods.

Research is being done on the raw food diet, but no studies have looked at the diet's effect on diabetes specifically. I would continue to cook my foods and watch for more research.

The Maker's Diet

The Maker's Diet is based on eating foods that God "intended," meaning eating whole natural foods, including organic meats, fruits, and vegetables. This is not just a diet; it includes lifestyle changes that help you strengthen the four pillars of health—physical, spiritual, mental, and emotional—including increasing physical activity, reducing stress, and finding faith. The diet claims to improve your health and promote weight loss, which will lower your risks for chronic illnesses including diabetes.

The diet is broken down into three phases—the first of which allows no carbohydrates. The next two phases slowly reintroduce healthy foods including whole grains, fruits, and vegetables and organic meats including beef and chicken.

The diet recommends a large number of supplements—items the author of the book happens to sell on his Website. He offers a membership that includes meal plans and advice. The author says that the diet is well researched in clinical trials and studies, but doesn't give evidence to prove this claim. Therefore, find faith on your own terms, eat well, and don't buy dozens of supplements that might cause more harm than good.

The Ayurvedic Diet

The ayurvedic diet, popularized by author and doctor Deepak Chopra, is based on a system of medicine that originated in ancient India. It attempts to balance and restore harmony in your body by using diet, yoga, and herbs. The diet is built on a theory that we are born with unique characteristics based on the combination of "doshas" in our gene structure. The doshas are dynamic forces within the universe including earth, water, fire, and wind. Ayurvedic doctors determine which doshas are strongest and which are out of balance, and give you a diet prescription that strengthens and balances them. Ayurvedic practitioners claim that this diet will bring harmony back to your body and, in doing so, help you meet your weight goals and decrease the likelihood of chronic illnesses including diabetes.

Many people using this diet say their health improves. Right now, no research has looked at ayurvedic diet alone; studies are examining some of the herbs used in ayurvedic medicine. If you eat appropriate varieties of food and the right fats, this diet can be a balanced one without excesses of saturated fat. You will need to find a good ayurvedic practitioner to guide you and it will take some time and commitment to change your diet completely.

Alternative Supplements

Even people who don't opt to make a complete diet change may incorporate alternative supplements as part of their nutritional intake and health-seeking lifestyle.

Ayurvedic Treatments

What is it and what does it do? Ayurvedic treatments are complicated because there is a long history and there are more than 1200 plants used in ayurvedic herbal preparations. Some of the herbs used in the treatment of diabetes include gymnema sylvestre, coccinia indica, fenugreek, holy dasil, D-400, and Ayush-82.

Does it work? The Department of Health and Human Services conducted a very large review of studies using these herbs in the treatment of diabetes.

So, are the benefits worth the risks? Many of the herbs were found to be beneficial but there is no evidence to suggest long term benefit from herbal preparations. If you want to try ayurvedic medicine and herbs, see a doctor who practices this form of medicine and be sure you talk to your diabetes dream team and keep them involved.

ALA (Alpha-lipoic Acid)

What is it and what does it do? ALA is a coenzyme—it works with another enzyme—to help our body metabolize carbohydrates. In diabetes treatment, this supplement is believed to lower blood sugar and treat neuropathy (nerve damage), and improve insulin resistance that is found in type 2 diabetes. It's also a powerful antioxidant which may help prevent heart disease and cancer. You can get ALA from foods including spinach, broccoli, potatoes, yeast, liver, and kidneys.

Does it work? Many studies are looking at the possible benefits of using this supplement to treat diabetes. It has been shown to improve neuropathy symptoms when given intravenously but not when taken orally; it improved insulin sensitivity and blood-sugar usage among people with type 2 diabetes when used both intravenously and orally.

So, are the benefits worth the risks? The numbness associated with neuropathy might get worse before it gets better. When taken intravenously, ALA might cause nausea, vomiting, and headache. Allergies to ALA have been reported, too. It might cause deficiencies of some nutrients like iron and thiamine. Alcohol also causes a decrease in the effectiveness of ALA. Because this drug can affect your blood sugar, you need to discuss this with your dream team. You may need adjustments in your medications.

Biotin

What is it and what does it do? Biotin is a B vitamin that helps metabolize protein, fat, and carbohydrates. It also helps another folic acid, another B vitamin, work. It might increase insulin secretion, which would lower blood-sugar levels.

Does it work? Studies suggest that when taken at a high dose (100 mcg a day) it might lower blood-sugar levels. This dose is much higher than the recommended daily dose of biotin (30 mcg a day). You could get biotin from foods such as egg yolks, milk, beef liver, yeast, and peanuts.

So, are the benefits worth the risks? Much like the other B vitamins, biotin is water-soluble which means that what you don't use you get rid of in your urine, so it's unlikely to cause problems. This vitamin might lower your blood sugar, so you should consult your doctor and other members of your dream team to talk about any possible need to lower your medication doses.

Carnitine

What is it and what does it do? Carnitine is an amino acid that helps the body use fat for energy. It is believed that carnitine can improve insulin sensitivity in people with type 2 diabetes. You can get it in foods such as meat and dairy.

Does it work? We still do not know. There is not enough research on carnitine supplementation and diabetes.

So, are the benefits worth the risks? Carnitine can cause nausea, vomiting, stomach cramps, heartburn, diarrhea, body odor, and seizures. People with liver disease or a seizure disorder like epilepsy should not take carnitine.

Chromium

What is it and what does it do? Chromium is an essential trace mineral; we need it in small amounts. Researchers believe that chromium helps blood sugar get into the cells. You can get chromium from foods such as yeast, whole grain cereals, broccoli, prunes, mushrooms, and beer.

Does it work? There is controversy about whether chromium works or not. Many studies have shown that chromium supplements can reduce trigylceride levels, lower blood sugar, and improve insulin levels. However, the government says there isn't enough evidence to support these claims.

So, are the benefits worth the risks? At low doses, supplementation with chromium appears to be safe, but most of the research hasn't looked at long-term use. In higher doses, there are some serious concerns. In high doses it can worsen kidney disease—a major problem for people with diabetes who already have an increased risk for kidney disease and kidney failure. For this reason alone, it's probably best to avoid chromium supplements.

Cinnamon

What is it and what does it do? Cinnamon is that familiar spice we've used for years in foods and beverages. It is currently unknown how cinnamon would improve blood-sugar control.

Does it work? Little research has been done to report one way or another; what has been done has produced conflicting results.

So, are the benefits worth the risks? Clearly, cinnamon in small amounts is safe, though some people are allergic to it. But little research has been done to determine the safety of consuming large amounts of cinnamon. If you want to try cinnamon, add a little to your morning tea or coffee, sprinkle on salads or oatmeal, or add it to the spices that coat your chicken. If it doesn't help your blood sugar it will enhance your meals by making your food taste good.

Co-Enzyme Q-10

What is it and what does it do? CoQ10 is an essential part of energy production. You need it to convert glucose (blood sugar) into energy. The theory is that if you consume more CoQ10, it will move glucose into the energy cycle and out of the blood.

Does it work? Currently, research in this area is conflicting—some studies find benefits while others don't. It's possible that the reason for mixed results is that some people might be CoQ10 deficient and, by providing it in the form of a supplement, you are giving the body what it needs. More research is needed before we'll know if it has benefits.

So, are the benefits worth the risks? When CoQ10 is used orally at low doses, it is generally safe, but it might cause nausea, diarrhea, and loss of appetite. However, some safety concerns exist specifically if you take the blood thinner coumadin (Warfarin), because CoQ10 can lower the effects of the medication.

Garlic

What is it and what does it do? Besides flavoring our food, garlic has been considered a medicinal plant for centuries. It has many claims including the ability to lower cholesterol levels, blood pressure and, possibly, blood sugar. The latter claim is because we know that garlic contains allicin, a component of allylpropyl disulfide, a substance known to reduce blood sugar and increase insulin in people who don't have diabetes.

Does it work? Only a few studies have evaluated this claim and those didn't find promising results.

So, are the benefits worth the risks? Garlic is definitely safe in the amounts found in foods, and possibly safe if appropriate amounts are taken orally as a supplement. However, there are some concerns that garlic can interact with some medications including those taken for HIV/AIDS, blood thinners, and birth control pills.

One clove of fresh garlic provides enough allicin to meet the typical dose found in most supplements. Cooking destroys most of the allicin found in the clove so to get the most benefit you need to consume garlic raw. If you use cooked garlic more than one clove a day will be needed to reach the typical dose.

Ginseng

What is it and what does it do? Ginseng is a family of plants, the roots of which contain active ingredients known as ginsenosides. The dried root is used to make pills, creams, or tea. The type of ginseng that appears to have the most potent actions is Asian ginseng, but its close relative American ginseng has similar properties. We don't know how ginseng works, but it does seem to lower blood glucose and hemoglobin A1C in people with diabetes not using insulin.

Does it work? Some studies suggest that ginseng does lower blood sugar. The problem is that the majority of the studies are small or flawed. A few large, well-designed studies have prompted the government to conduct additional research studies on ginseng and diabetes.

So, are the benefits worth the risks? Ginseng has been found to be generally safe to use for up to three months. After that, unpleasant reactions may occur. Some of the side effects of Asian ginseng include insomnia, headaches, vertigo, palpitations, and stomach upset. It can increase blood pressure, which can be especially dangerous if you have hypertension. Taking ginseng and using caffeine can raise your heart rate and blood pressure. It also interacts with blood thinners and could increase your risk of bleeding. And because it's possible for ginseng to lower blood sugar, if you are taking diabetes medications you could experience hypoglycemia, low blood sugar. Make sure that you discuss using ginseng with your doctor and all the other members on your team.

Inositol

What is it and what does it do? Inositol is an important part of cell membranes, and allows fat out of the liver and intestinal cells. Some believe this supplement can reduce the symptoms of diabetic neuropathy.

Does it work? Studies suggest that this supplement doesn't reduce the symptoms of diabetic nerve damage.

So, are the benefits worth the risks? The use of inositol is most likely safe, but because the probability that it will work is so low it doesn't make sense to take it.

Magnesium

What is it and what does it do? Magnesium is a mineral that is involved in more than 300 cellular functions in the body. Research suggests that if you have a magnesium deficiency, your body may be less sensitive to insulin. This has led to the use of magnesium supplements for type 2 diabetes.

Does it work? There are benefits when used orally and in appropriate amounts (400 mg daily but no more than 600 mg daily).

So, are the benefits worth the risks? Larger amounts of magnesium can cause nausea, vomiting, diarrhea; extreme amounts of magnesium can be serious and fatal. Symptoms include low blood pressure, muscle weakness, slowed breathing, coma, and heart failure. Magnesium can also interact with medications such as some antibiotics and water pills.

Potassium

What is it and what does it do? Potassium is a mineral that plays a role in balancing your blood and body pH. It also functions in other physiological processes such as transmission of nerve impulses, muscle contraction, kidney function, tissue production, and the production of carbohydrates. It might improve insulin resistance, though we don't know why. You can find potassium naturally in many foods such as fruits (bananas, kiwi, oranges), cereals, beans, milk, and vegetables.

Does it work? There isn't enough information for us to make a statement about potassium's ability to improve insulin resistance.

So, are the benefits worth the risks? Potassium is most likely safe if consumed in normal amounts—3,500 mg per day, including what you get in your diet. In large amounts, potassium supplementation can be fatal. If you have problems with your kidneys you may need to restrict potassium. Talk to your health care provider to determine how much potassium is right for you.

Vanadium

What is it and what does it do? Vanadium is a trace mineral that seems to be important in many enzyme reactions. Some believe that vanadium might be able to mimic the effects of insulin. Researchers think that vanadium turns on the receptor that allows glucose into the cells, and encourages the storage of carbohydrates in the liver and muscles while preventing the liver from making glucose. Therefore, the claim is that it both lowers blood glucose levels and increases insulin sensitivity in type 2 diabetes, but not in type 1 diabetes. It can be found in milk, seafood, oils, cereals, and vegetables.

Does it work? There is some research to suggest that it does both, reduce blood glucose levels and improve insulin sensitivity, but this seems to be the case only in individuals who don't need insulin.

So, are the benefits worth the risks? In small amounts, it seems safe enough. In larger doses, side effects include stomach problems like diarrhea, renal disease, and even death. I would hold off on vanadium or try to get it from your foods.

Vitamin B12

What is it and what does it do? Vitamin B12, also known as cobalamin, has many functions including the production of nerve cells. This may be the origin of the claim that B12 improves nerve damage in diabetes patients.

Does it work? Unfortunately, not enough research has looked at this B vitamin to make a statement in support or against this claim.

So, are the benefits worth the risks? Vitamin B12 is considered safe if you have a B12 deficiency. When taken orally, it can cause diarrhea and itching. You can get B12 in your diet by consuming foods such as meat, fish, and dairy products.

Many supplements claim to help people with diabetes, but very few have been able to truly show a benefit. Research continues. In the mean time you can get many of these supplements safely through your diet.

Power Points

🖝 A healthy diet is one that helps to maintain or improve your health and includes fresh fruits, vegetables, whole grains, non fat dairy, meat, poultry, and fish.

🖝 There is no clear evidence that people with diabetes who do not have vitamin or mineral deficiencies will benefit from supplementation.

🖝 Talk to your diabetes dream team about any herbs or supplements you are taking. You want to make sure that any supplement you take doesn't interact negatively with your medication.

🖝 Keep a list of the supplements and herbs you are taking along with the dosage. Bring the list with you when visiting members of your diabetes dream team.

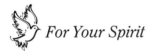 *For Your Spirit*

The Wise Ones

They thought he was crazy. Who in his right mind would suggest that the way to end your mistreatment by a group of people would be to sit down beside them at their lunch counters and on their buses? Who would suggest that walking—just walking, arm in arm, singing hymns—would be a better way to bring a nation to consciousness and conscience than waging a bloody battle? But, inspired by Gandhi, who did a similar thing in India, it's what Martin Luther King did.

Our greatest spiritual and moral leaders—Jesus first among them—didn't follow the status quo, but offered a radical brand of change. They knew that the same old approach would beget the same old result, so they dreamed up innovative approaches to accomplishing their goals. Their audacity usually succeeded—proof that there is more than one way to skin a...situation.

The same is true in our lives. It's easy to follow the well-worn path we seem to have been set on, but when we want something new in our lives, we have to *do* something new. When we want change, we have to change. That is true whether you are trying to change the world, or change your glucose meter reading.

Change what? Change how? You can answer those questions by first going within, through prayer and meditation, to discover what is true and right for you. Then by opening your heart and mind to the infinite possibilities from which to choose your approach. And finally by releasing your fears long enough to take radical action—whatever radical may mean to you. You have to summon your faith, too. Believe that you will be able to accomplish what you set out to do. Even if everyone thinks you're crazy.

10 How Much Is "A Little Sugar"? Monitoring Your Glucose

Before the early 1970s, controlling your blood glucose required a lot of guesswork. Urine testing was the only method of measuring glucose levels—and it was highly inaccurate and had many limitations. In fact, it couldn't really tell you what you glucose levels were—just that, if there was glucose in your urine, the level in your blood was *way* too high.

In the 1960s, a company called Ames R&D developed a way to test blood directly. You put a drop of blood on a thin paper strip, let it sit for a minute, then washed it off. The strip would turn a shade of blue that gave you an estimate of your blood glucose. They were not easy to read; they were easy to misinterpret. So a scientist invented a machine that could read the test more accurately—and even give you a specific number based on the exact shade of blue on the test strip. With that, the first glucose meter was born.

After the patent for it was issued in 1971 and blood glucose monitoring became more popular in the 80s, urine testing went out the window, except to test for ketones and the protein albumin in urine, both of which indicate problems with diabetes control. Many changes have occurred that have made meters easier to use, with features that make them better tools at monitoring your blood glucose levels and trends. It's an important part of diabetes management, and will become an essential aspect of your lifestyle.

SMBG

The process of monitoring your own blood glucose is called self monitoring of blood glucose (SMBG). To SMBG, you need testing strips, a lancing device, and a glucose meter.

The Test Strips

In general, the test strip is plastic with a small area that contains a chemical that reacts with glucose in the blood. The main difference in test strips lies in how they accept your blood sample. The "capillary fill" strips suck blood into the strip through capillary action; it's more hygienic and less likely to contaminate the machine. "Top dosing" strips require you to apply the blood to the test strip either inside or outside the machine. Different types of meters read your glucose levels in different ways. You'll need to know which strips are compatible to your unit. (More on this follows.)

Proper storage and handling of test strips is essential for accurate results. Never use the test strips after the expiration date, and once the box has been opened, toss unused strips after four months, regardless of the date on the box. Don't bend or cut the strips. Because the strips are sensitive to moisture and light, store them in their original moisture-resistant and light-protected vial. Keep them away from direct sunlight and heat, but don't put them in the fridge. Toss a strip after you use it, of course.

The Lancet Device

A lancet device looks a little like a pen, but it contains a sharp, spring-loaded blade or needle inside. You use it to prick the skin to get the blood sample that goes on the test strip. It makes getting a blood sample quick and fairly painless.

To use it, first prepare everything you will need (test strip, lancet, glucose meter). Wash your hands with soap and warm water and dry them completely. This will help prevent an infection at the puncture site and eliminate the possibility of contaminating the blood sample with glucose from food that you might have touched. It also warms your hands, which makes the blood flow more easily. We no longer recommend using an alcohol swab to clean your hands because alcohol can gradually dry your skin causing cracks and calluses which can lead to infection.

To obtain the blood sample hold the lancet device against your skin—usually on the side of your fingertip—and press the button to release the lancet. It is not recommended to use the center of your fingertip; there are more nerve endings there which will cause it to hurt more. You can control how deep the puncture goes by adjusting how hard you press your finger against the device: press hard for a deeper prick. Most devices also come with different lancet covers that allow you to adjust how deep the lancet will penetrate. A thicker cover won't let the lancet plunge too far into soft or thin skin, areas of the hand that aren't as fleshy, or children's tender finders. The other cover is meant for thick or calloused skin. Many lancet devices have numbers which allow you to set the device for depth control. Your goal is to get the puncture deep enough that you get an adequate amount of blood for the test but not so deep that you cause pain and bruising.

Once you have made the puncture, hold your hand down and squeeze your finger using rhythmic motions until a small amount of blood appears. How much blood you will need depends on the type of strip you use. Strips that require top dosing may require a large drop of blood, a small drop for test strips that have capillary action. Apply the blood to the test strip and follow the directions for the glucose meter.

Often, lancing devices are included in the blood glucose monitoring kits, but they are generally inexpensive. Invest in another one; it's always useful to have a spare. Never borrow one or share yours with anyone because there is a risk of transmitting disease.

Reset the lancet for the next use. Some lancets have a simple mechanism that you can push or pull to reset the spring loader. Others require you to remove the cover so that the lancet can be pushed back into the starting position.

New products are being introduced that make using glucose meters easier. For instance, there is a laser skin perforator that makes a small hole in your fingertip without a lancet. It works by generating a single pulse of laser light. Currently this type of lancing device is available by prescription only.

The Meter

Generally, meters work one of two ways. In both types, the test strip contains a chemical that reacts to the glucose in the blood sample. The glucose reacts with the chemical causing the pH (amount of acid) in the blood to change the color of the indicator on the strip.

Photometric meters, the most commonly used kind, read the color on the glucose strip and compare it to the meter's internal components. The amount of color change is translated into a glucose number. The amperometric meter measures the change in pH by measuring the voltage changes in the electrical charge that passes through the blood sample.

There are more than 25 different types of meters on the market with a variety of different features.

▶ Audio meters allow people with visual impairment (a common complication of diabetes) to check their own blood glucose. This meter gives verbal instructions that direct the tester through the process from start to finish. Then it tells you your blood glucose result. These sophisticated meters even speak several different languages.

▶ Alternate test site meters let individuals obtain their blood sample from an area other than their fingertip. You've probably seen B. B. King promoting the One Touch Ultra System that allows for forearm testing. In the ad, he talks about the importance of being able to preserve his fingers for his guitar playing. The fingertip and forearm provide similar results when you're testing fasting blood glucose, but there seems to be a difference in results taken after a meal. Then the fingertip blood sample is higher than the forearm measure. Other studies have found a difference in how alternate test site meters capture results when blood glucose is low. If you feel symptoms of low blood glucose, test your finger instead of your forearm. Or rub or tap your forearm before you do the test; more consistent results are likely.

▶ Data management systems are software packages that make tracking your blood glucose easier by automatically recording the data from each blood test. Some of the data management systems are actually part of the meter so that everything is in one unit. If your meter doesn't come with the system, make sure that your meter is compatible with any software you buy. Because some of the software is more difficult to use, test-drive the software before buying. And the software is an extra, not a necessity; if you can't afford it or won't use it, don't bother.

▶ Continuous glucose monitors are different from the traditional meters in that they allow you to get readings every few minutes around the clock. This permits you to keep track of problems and helps you make appropriate adjustments throughout the day. They also have an alarm that will let you know when your blood glucose is going too high or too low. This monitor works by sampling the fluid around your cells (interstitial fluid) obtained by a small catheter placed just under the skin. This technology is so new that experts are suggesting that results should be double-checked using a traditional meter.

Recommendations for Frequency of Use

Generally, blood glucose should be monitored two to four times a day, either before meals or two hours after meals and at bedtime. But each case is unique; you may need to test more frequently:

▹ If you are having problems with low or high blood glucose.

▹ To understand how food, medicine, and exercise affect your blood glucose.

▹ When your diabetes medications are changed.

> ⊳ If you are prescribed new medications (including those that are not for diabetes).

> ⊳ When you become sick or are recovering from an illness.

> ⊳ When you have increased levels of stress (i.e. you are going through a divorce).

> ⊳ When you change your activity level.

> ⊳ If you take insulin or are on an insulin pump.

> ⊳ If you are pregnant or are planning to be.

The results of your test can help you manage your diabetes day-by-day or even hour-by-hour.

You and your dream team need to use both the SMBG and the A1C test to get a complete picture of your blood glucose control. The A1C test tells you what your average blood glucose level has been every day for the past 90 days. It's the best way to know your overall blood-glucose control during this period of time. The higher your A1C results, the higher the amount of glucose in your blood and the greater your chances are for serious health problems.

Your A1C test results are reported in percentage points and your SMBG results are measured in milligrams per deciliter (mg/dl). If you're like many people with diabetes, you found it very difficult to correlate the two measures. Now the American Diabetes Association has given your dream team a way to report both test using the same unit of measure—mg/dl. It's called estimated average glucose (eAG) and it's calculated from your A1C test.

The chart on page 126 identifies the guidelines set by the American College of Endocrinology (ACE) and the American Diabetes Association (ADA) for optimal blood glucose control to prevent diabetes complications. Again, diabetes is unique to each patient, so your individual goals should be set with your dream team, and you should work with them closely to adjust your diabetes care plan if you aren't meeting those objectives.

Most people think that food is the only factor that needs to be adjusted when you're trying to achieve glucose control. Yes, food may be of primary concern if you are overeating. But if you maintain a well-balanced, low-calorie diet, and you're still not meeting your target glucose levels, you may need to change the timing or type of your diabetes medication. You may also benefit from an increase in your physical activity, or a change in the timing or type of exercise you do. Additionally, a change in how you distribute your carbs throughout your meals on a given day may help as well.

Optimal Glucose Control

ADA	ACE

A1C scores
    less than 7.0% (eAG** 154 mg/dl)   less than 6.5% (eAG 140 mg/dl)
Fasting glucose*
    90-130 mg/dl   less than 110 mg/dl
2-hour post meal glucose
    less than 180 mg/dl at peak   less than140 mg/dl
*Fasting blood glucose is taken first thing in the morning, before eating.
**Estimated average glucose calculated from A1C scores.

Blood Glucose Records

Keeping track of your SMBG results—and making note of what was going on in your life at the time—will help you identify how food, activity, stress, and medication affect your glucose levels. A glucose record chart can help you monitor your results, your meals, your activities, and your moods. It seems like just one more extra thing to add to your schedule, but through time you'll see the benefit in taking time to examine your habits this way. The more accurate you are in your blood glucose record the more successful you will be in managing your diabetes. The following is a chart that shows you how to keep thorough blood glucose records. Your record should include:

- What kinds of foods are eaten.
- How much food is eaten, include preparation method, and ingredient lists for mixed dishes such as salad.
- What kinds of beverages you drink. (Note if you use sugar or artificial sweetener, caffeinated or decaffeinated.)
- Carbohydrate value of the food, determined by counting grams of carbohydrate or carbohydrate choices.
- Timing of meals.
- Diabetes medication—how much and what time.
- Blood glucose readings before and after meals.
- Physical activity—what kind, how much, and when.
- Comments—feelings of high or low blood glucose.

Sample Blood Glucose Record

DAILY FOOD/SMBG DIARY		FIRST DAY Monday	DATE 3/26	SECOND DAY Tuesday	DATE 3/27

MEAL	FOOD CHOICE/ SERVING SIZE	FOOD GROUP	CARB CHOICE/ GRAMS	MEDICATION	SMBG / COMMENTS	
					TIME	BG
BREAKFAST	Café' au lait - 1/2 c milk, 1/2 c coffee, 1 Splenda	1/2 milk	6 grams	850 mg metformin	Before	100
	1/2 vanilla yogurt, non-fat	1/2 milk	6 grams		2 hr After	120
	1/2 c chopped fresh mango	1 fruit	15 grams			
	1/2 c yellow grits	1 grain	15 grams			
SNACK						
LUNCH	2 slices whole grain bread	2 grain	30 grams		Before	100
	2 oz turkey breast	2 lean meat	0 grams			
	1 tsp mayo	1 fat	0 grams		2 hr After	110
	1 peach	1 fruit	15 grams			
	water					
DINNER	1 c pole beans	2 vegetable	8 grams	850 mg metformin	Before	140
	2 dumplings	2 grain	30 grams			
	4 oz chicken breast, no skin	4 lean meat	0 grams		2 hr After	135
	1/4 cup brown gravy	1/2 grain	8 grams			
	diet ice tea					
SNACK	1 cup buttermilk	1 milk	15 grams			140
	5 triscuits	1 grain	15 grams			
	1 oz low-fat Colby cheese	1 lean meat	0 grams			

Once you complete your blood glucose record, you are ready to look for patterns that can help you make adjustments in your food, activity, or medication. First, look for blood glucose numbers that do not meet your target range, whether it's above or below your target. Circle high and low readings in different colors. Then ask yourself the following questions to help you identify and solve the problem.

- ▷ Did you measure your food portions?
- ▷ Were your food portions smaller or larger than usual?
- ▷ Did you eat more or less carbohydrate than usual?
- ▷ Did you forget to take your diabetes medication?
- ▷ Have you increased or decreased your diabetes medication?
- ▷ Were you more or less active than usual?
- ▷ Are you under stress or sick?
- ▷ Did you start taking over-the-counter medication or an herbal supplement?
- ▷ Did you drink alcohol without eating?

Once you've identified the problem, look at some solutions.

For high blood glucose readings:
- ▷ Use measuring spoons, cups, and food scales to get accurate portions.
- ▷ Eat less total carbohydrate at meals.
- ▷ Take medication as prescribed. Write yourself a reminder and put it where you'll notice it.
- ▷ Talk with a member of your diabetes dream team about making changes in your medication dose.
- ▷ Increase your daily activity,
- ▷ Discuss over-the-counter-medications and herbal supplements with a member of your diabetes dream team.

For low blood glucose readings:
- ▷ Use measuring spoons, cups and food scales to get accurate portions.
- ▷ Eat enough carbohydrate at meals.

> ▹ Take medication as prescribed.

> ▹ Eat extra carbs if you are going to be more active. You may also need to take less medication—your diabetes dream team can help here.

> ▹ Do not drink alcohol without eating. Have a small meal or snack before drinking. Limit alcohol to 1 to 2 drinks per day.

Because controlling your blood-sugar levels lowers your risk of diabetes complications, knowing your blood sugar gives you the best defense against diabetes. Make copies of the blank blood glucose record at the end of this chapter and use it daily to help manage your diabetes. Bring your blood glucose record and meter with you when you visit any member of your diabetes dream team so you can talk about reaching your blood glucose goals.

Power Points

☞ Urine tests for glucose are inaccurate and are no longer recommended.

☞ The process of monitoring your blood glucose is called self monitoring of blood glucose (SMBG).

☞ To monitor your glucose you need a testing strip, lancing device, and meter.

☞ Wash your hands with warm soapy water before SMBG.

☞ Generally, blood glucose should be monitored two to four times a day, either before meals or two hours after meals and at bedtime.

☞ The A1C test and SMBG give you and your diabetes dream team a complete picture of your blood glucose control. Optimal glucose levels are:

Before meals	90 to 130
1 to 2 hours after meals	less than 180
A1C	less than 7

☞ Keeping track of your SMBG results help you identify how food, activity, stress, and medication affect your glucose levels.

Daily Food/SMBG Diary

DAILY FOOD/SMBG DIARY   FIRST DAY   DATE

MEAL	FOOD CHOICE/ SERVING SIZE	FOOD GROUP	CARB CHOICE/ GRAMS	MEDICATION	SMBG / COMMENTS	
BREAKFAST					TIME Before 2 hr After	BG
SNACK						
LUNCH					Before 2 hr After	
DINNER					Before 2 hr After	
SNACK						

Day 2 Daily Food/SMBG Diary

DAILY FOOD/SMBG DIARY   SECOND DAY   DATE

MEAL	FOOD CHOICE/ SERVING SIZE	FOOD GROUP	CARB CHOICE/ GRAMS	MEDICATION	SMBG / COMMENTS	
BREAKFAST					TIME Before 2 hr After	BG
SNACK						
LUNCH					Before 2 hr After	
DINNER					Before 2 hr After	
SNACK						

© 2005 CBR Nutrition Enterprises

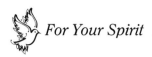 *For Your Spirit*

Excuses, Excuses

You missed the deadline on that project at work. You forgot to send your best friend a birthday card. You were driving just a *little bit* over the speed limit. When we haven't done something we're supposed to do, excuses come easily. We use them to justify our failure or avoid blame.

Consider a person with diabetes who insists that he can't self-monitor blood glucose because he doesn't know how. That may be an excuse. But it may also be an explanation—and there is a difference.

An explanation takes into account the underlying reasons that a person can't do something. If you go off your diet because you couldn't pass by the "hot doughnuts" sign in the bakery window, that's an excuse. You're not focused on the actual problem. (Why can't you resist the bakery?) But if you know that you tend to overeat because of depression, you are offering an explanation. You're not saying that you can't lose weight; you are just describing the obstacle that you have to overcome. And then, if you seek counseling to deal with the depression, you are actively accepting personal responsibility for overcoming that obstacle.

The difference is subtle. And it has less to do with the particular circumstances, and more to do with your ability to look within for the things that are stopping you and to find the motivation to work through them. Are you willing to go beyond the apparent reason something isn't going the way it should to get to the real reason for the obstacle? And then are you willing to do the work—whatever it takes—to overcome it?

Take that person with the glucose monitor. He may honestly not know how to use the monitor. Maybe he didn't get good instruction from his doctor; maybe the directions that came with the monitor weren't clear. But if he's motivated to learn, he can consult with someone on his dream team for instructions or ask a friend to help him translate the written instructions.

Excuses are easier. But they deny you the opportunity to tap into your personal power and spiritual strength, to be accountable for your actions and to see yourself truly succeed.

11 Weighing in on Diabetes and Dieting

What shape do you think you're in? If you are like many African-Americans, your perception of healthy weight may be different from what other folks think. There are many cultural factors that effect ones perception of weight and body image. Some years ago, Sir Mix-A-Lot rapped in his wildly popular song Baby Got Back, "I like big butts and I cannot lie." By traditional western standards, a narrow, flat behind is ideal, but from the black man's view, a beautiful body is defined by some heft and some hips. A 1994 article in Ebony magazine describes this sentiment from a brother's perspective. In the article "When Bigger is Better: Men who Like Big Women," one bachelor said he likes a "woman of size"—a term he preferred to "overweight" or "heavy." Other terms we use to describe large folks include "big-boned," "thick," "full figured," or "phat."

It's not just men who think bigger is better. Culturally, most sisters do not perceive being overweight with being unattractive, and research shows that even teenage girls—the population perhaps most obsessed with body image and looks—don't think being pretty is defined by being skinny. That's good news for our self-esteem—but not so great for our health.

If having some meat on your bones is desirable and being "thick" is positive, you may not consider yourself overweight if you're heavier than the norm. In a recent survey, more than half of the African-Americans who were clinically overweight and about a quarter of those who were obese believed that their weight was normal. If you don't know you are overweight, why would you try to lose weight? Well the answer, of course, is that you wouldn't.

But when it comes to your health what you don't know can hurt you. As a matter of fact, weight loss is one of the best ways to manage your diabetes. Losing as little as 10 to 15 pounds is enough to improve blood glucose levels. Weight loss can also decrease insulin resistance, which means your pancreas won't need to work as hard to produce insulin and less insulin will be needed to control blood glucose. This will help your pancreas to last longer and you may be able to decrease the amount of oral diabetes medication and/or insulin needed to control your blood glucose. Weight loss can also improve blood cholesterol and triglyceride levels, improve blood pressure, and help you to live longer with a better quality of life.

So What Shape Are You Really In?

There are two common reasons for being overweight—eating too much and not being active enough. Yes, there are folks with thyroid conditions or other health concerns, but for most of us it's just a matter of too little exercise and too much "diet." If you eat more calories than your body burns, the extra calories are stored as fat. We all need a little fat to cushion the body's frame and protect our organs. But too much fat results in being overweight.

Where your fat is located can also indicate health problems. If your fat is located in the abdominal area—you're shaped like an apple—you are at greater risk for heart disease. That's also an indicator that you might have insulin resistance. When you reduce the amount of fat in the stomach area you can improve insulin resistance and diabetes control. If you are shaped like a pear—your fat is located in the hips and thighs—your risk for heart disease is less. Waist measurements more than 40 inches for men and 35 inches for women are indicators of increased risk for heart disease and high blood pressure.

Body Mass Index (BMI) is another measurement that helps to assess your weight and risk for disease and death. BMI is a measure of your weight in relation to your height and is used as an estimate of your body fat. Combining the BMI and waist measurement will tell you your risk for developing other obesity associated disease.

What Is Your Risk?

Obesity increases the risk for a number of diseases including diabetes. It also makes it more difficult to manage some diseases—including diabetes. The following steps will help you find out your obesity disease risk:

Use the BMI tables shown on pages 135–136 to estimate your total body fat. Locate your height in the left hand column and read across the row for that height to your body weight. The height in the chart is listed as inches. So, you will need to convert your height into inches first.

Body Mass Index Chart

BMI	19	20	21	22	23	24	25	26	27	28	29	30	31	32	33	34	35
Height (inches)							Body Weight (pounds)										
58	91	96	100	105	110	115	119	124	129	134	138	143	148	153	158	162	167
59	94	99	104	109	114	119	124	128	133	138	143	148	153	158	163	168	173
60	97	102	107	112	118	123	128	133	138	143	148	153	158	163	168	174	179
61	100	106	111	116	122	127	132	137	143	148	153	158	164	169	174	180	185
62	104	109	115	120	126	131	136	142	147	153	158	164	169	175	180	186	191
63	107	113	118	124	130	135	141	146	152	158	163	169	175	180	186	191	197
64	110	116	122	128	134	140	145	151	157	163	169	174	180	186	192	197	204
65	114	120	126	132	138	144	150	156	162	168	174	180	186	192	198	204	210
66	118	124	130	136	142	148	155	161	167	173	179	186	192	198	204	210	216
67	121	127	134	140	146	153	159	166	172	178	185	191	198	204	211	217	223
68	125	131	138	144	151	158	164	171	177	184	190	197	203	210	216	223	230
69	128	135	142	149	155	162	169	176	182	189	196	203	209	216	223	230	236
70	132	139	146	153	160	167	174	181	188	195	202	209	216	222	229	236	243
71	136	143	150	157	165	172	179	186	193	200	208	215	222	229	236	243	250
72	140	147	154	162	169	177	184	191	199	206	213	221	228	235	242	250	258
73	144	151	159	166	174	182	189	197	204	212	219	227	235	242	250	257	265
74	148	155	163	171	179	186	194	202	210	218	225	233	241	249	256	264	272
75	152	160	168	176	184	192	200	208	216	224	232	240	248	256	264	272	279
76	156	164	172	180	189	197	205	213	221	230	238	246	254	263	271	279	287

Body Mass Index Chart (page 2)

BMI	36	37	38	39	40	41	42	43	44	45	46	47	48	49	50	51	52	53	54
Height (inches)	Body Weight (pounds)																		
58	172	177	181	186	191	196	201	205	210	215	220	224	229	234	239	244	248	253	258
59	178	183	188	193	198	203	208	212	217	222	227	232	237	242	247	252	257	262	267
60	184	189	194	199	204	209	215	220	225	230	235	240	245	250	255	261	266	271	276
61	190	195	201	206	211	217	222	227	232	238	243	248	254	259	264	269	275	280	285
62	196	202	207	213	218	224	229	235	240	246	251	256	262	267	273	278	284	289	295
63	203	208	214	220	225	231	237	242	248	254	259	265	270	278	282	287	293	299	304
64	209	215	221	227	232	238	244	250	256	262	267	273	279	285	291	296	302	308	314
65	216	222	228	234	240	246	252	258	264	270	276	282	288	294	300	306	312	318	324
66	223	229	235	241	247	253	260	266	272	278	284	291	297	303	309	315	322	328	334
67	230	236	242	249	255	261	268	274	280	287	293	299	306	312	319	325	331	338	344
68	236	243	249	256	262	269	276	282	289	295	302	308	315	322	328	335	341	348	354
69	243	250	257	263	270	277	284	291	297	304	311	318	324	331	338	345	351	358	365
70	250	257	264	271	278	285	292	299	306	313	320	327	334	341	348	355	362	369	376
71	257	265	272	279	286	293	301	308	315	322	329	338	343	351	358	365	372	379	386
72	265	272	279	287	294	302	309	316	324	331	338	346	353	361	368	375	383	390	397
73	272	280	288	295	302	310	318	325	333	340	348	355	363	371	378	386	393	401	408
74	280	287	295	303	311	319	326	334	342	350	358	365	373	381	389	396	404	412	420
75	287	295	303	311	319	327	335	343	351	359	367	375	383	391	399	407	415	423	431
76	295	304	312	320	328	336	344	353	361	369	377	385	394	402	410	418	426	435	443

From: http://www.nhlbisupport.com/bmi/bmicalc.htm

- Multiply the number of feet by 12 and then add the remaining inches. You use 12 because there are 12 inches in one foot.

Example: Say you are 5 feet 6 inches tall:

Multiply 5 × 12 = 60 inches

Then add the remaining 6 inches

60 inches + 6 inches = 66 inches

- Follow the column of your weight up to the top row that lists the BMI. Using the example above let's say you are 66 inches tall and weigh 186 pounds. Your BMI would be 30.

Write your BMI here _____

The BMI scores mean the following;

Below 18.5	Underweight
18.5 – 24.9	Normal
25.0 – 29.9	Overweight
30.0 – 39.9	Obesity
40.0 and above	Morbid Obesity

What does your score tell you about your weight?

I am _____

- Measure your waist by placing a measuring tape snugly around your waist where your belly button is.

What is your waist size? _____

- Now with your BMI and waist size determined, use the following table shown on page 138 to determine your health risk relative to normal weight.

Risk of Associated Disease According to BMI and Waist Size

BMI		Waist less than or equal to 40 in. (men) or 35 in. (women)	Waist greater than 40 in. (men) or 35 in. (women)
18.5 or less	Underweight	——	N/A
18.5 - 24.9	Normal	——	N/A
25.0 - 29.9	Overweight	Increased	High
30.0 - 34.9	Obese	High	Very High
35.0 - 39.9	Obese	Very High	Very High
40 or greater	Extremely Obese	Extremely High	Extremely High

From: http://www.nhlbi.nih.gov/healthpublic/heart/obesity/lose_wt/bmi_dis.htm

You should lose weight if you are obese (BMI greater than or equal to 30) or overweight (BMI of 25 to 29.9) and have two or more of the following risk factors:

High blood pressure (hypertension)

High LDL – cholesterol ("bad" cholesterol)

Low HDL – cholesterol ("good" cholesterol)

High triglycerides

High blood glucose (sugar)

Family history of premature heart disease

Physical inactivity

Cigarette smoking

How Much to Shed

If you need to lose weight, a slow gradual weight loss of half a pound to one pound weekly is the best weight-loss rate. Use the following formula to determine your daily calorie needs to promote weight loss. Be sure to discuss your weight loss goals with your diabetes dream team.

Use the BMI chart to determine what your weight would be if your BMI was less than 25. If that weight is unrealistic for you then set a more realistic weight. Keep in mind losing as little as 10–15 pounds is enough to improve blood glucose levels and your health.

- Multiply your goal weight by eleven.

  Goal weight × 11 = _____

  (Generally adults require 10 to 12 calories per pound of body weight. So, we use 11 to capture the mid range.)

  Let's say you want to weigh 150 pounds.

  150 × 11 = 1,650 calories

- If you are moderately active add 20% of calories to the total in line 2.

  (Line 2 × .20 = _____) + Line 2 = _____

  1,650 × .20 = 330 calories

  1,650 calories + 330 calories = 1980 total calories

  To promote weight loss you will need to subtract 500 calories from the above total.

  1,980 – 500 = 1,480 total calories for weight loss.

  If you desire weight gain add 500 calories to the above total.

- If you are very active add 40% of calories to the total in line 2.

  (Line 2 × .40 = _____) + Line 2 = _____

  1, 650 × .40 = 660

  1,650 calories + 660 calories = 2,310 total calories

  To promote weight loss you will need to subtract 500 calories from the above total.

  2,310 – 500 = 1,810 total calories for weight loss.

My goal weight is _____

My daily calorie requirement is _____

The following table can be used as a guide in your daily meal planning. It provides you with the number of daily servings from each food group based on your calorie needs. To achieve your weight goals, chose a calorie level that is close to your daily calorie requirement. Follow the column of your calorie level down to determine the number of daily servings you need from each food group.

Sample Meal Patterns					
Calories per day	1200	1500	1800	2000	2500
Daily servings from each food group					
Starch	5	7	8	9	11
Fruit	3	3	4	4	6
Milk	2	2	3	3	3
Vegetables	2	2	3	3	5
Meat/Meat Substitutes	4	4	6	6	8
Fat	3	4	4	5	6

You'll remember from the chapter on food pyramids that a single serving might include half a cup of grits, a third of a cup of rice, a medium apple. A cup of milk, half a cup cooked vegetables, an egg or an ounce of cheese or fish is also a serving. See page 141 for a more complete list.

There are perhaps a thousand different weight-loss plans out there— maybe more. But the key to all of them hinges on this fact: to lose weight you simply need to eat less than you usually do. So, if you need to lose weight, work on changing your portion sizes first.

What is a portion? Most people are confused when it comes to portions and servings, using the terms interchangeably. The fact is, portions and servings are two different measurements.

A portion is the amount of each food you *choose* to eat. A serving describes the amount of food *recommended* from each food group. It's the amount of food listed on the Nutrition Facts panel on packaged food or the amount of food recommended in MyPyramid and the Dietary Guidelines for Americans. Portions, of course, can be bigger or smaller than the recommended food servings. And if you're overweight and not losing pounds, its likely that your portions are larger than recommended serving sizes. You should first look at making sure your portion sizes are closer to standard serving sizes. The chart below provides a number of ways you can "guesstimate" your servings.

Serving Size Guide	
One Serving of ...	Looks Like a ...
Grain/Starch Products	
1 cup of cereal flakes	closed fist
1 pancake	compact disc
1/2 cup of cooked potato	1/2 baseball
1/3 cup rice or pasta	1 lemon
1 slice of bread	cassette tape
1 piece of corn bread	bar of soap
1/2 cup beans	1/2 baseball
4 small cookies	4 casino chips
Vegetables and Fruit	
1 cup of salad greens	baseball
1/2 cup cooked vegetables	1/2 baseball
1 baked potato	closed fist
1 med fruit	baseball
1/4 cup of raisins	large egg
Dairy and Cheese	
1 1/2 oz. cheese	4 stacked dice or a C battery
1/2 cup of ice cream	1/2 baseball
Meat and Alternatives	
3 oz. meat, fish, and poultry	deck of cards
3 oz. grilled/baked fish	checkbook
2 Tbsp. peanut butter	ping-pong ball or roll of film
Fats	
1 tsp. margarine or spreads	1 thumb tip
1 Tbsp. salad dressing	1 whole thumb

Using the plate method can help determine how much of a food to eat. Remember to make half your plate with a non-starchy vegetable, a quarter with a grain or starchy vegetable, and the other quarter with meat. But to control your portion size, change your plate size. If you usually use a 12-inch dinner plate try using a 9-inch dinner plate instead—and don't go back for seconds.

Diabetes and Dieting Myths

Myth: High-protein/low-carbohydrate diets are a healthy way to lose weight.

Fact: The long-term health effects of a high-protein/low-carbohydrate diet are unknown. But getting most of your daily calories from high-protein foods like meat, eggs, and cheese is not a balanced eating plan, and eating lots of those foods may mean you're eating too much fat and cholesterol, which may raise heart disease risk. You may be eating too few fruits, vegetables, and whole grains which give you the fiber you need to avoid constipation. And the diet may make you feel nauseous, tired, and weak. Eating fewer than 130 grams of carbohydrate a day can lead to the buildup of ketones—partially broken down fats—in your blood. A buildup of these in your blood (called ketosis) can cause your body to produce high levels of uric acid, which is a risk factor for kidney stones and gout, a painful swelling of the joints. Additionally, high-protein diets make the kidneys work harder and can worsen existing kidney disease.

Myth: Starches are fattening. Knock off the bread and rice when you're trying to lose weight.

Fact: Many high-starch foods like bread, rice, pasta, cereals, beans, fruits, and some vegetables (like potatoes and yams) are low in fat and calories—in their natural state. The fat and calories start to add up when you eat them in large portions or cover them with high-fat toppings such as butter, sour cream, or mayonnaise. Foods high in starch (also called complex carbohydrates) are an important source of energy for your body.

Myth: Certain foods such as grapefruit, celery, or cabbage soup, can burn fat and make you lose weight.

Fact: No foods can burn fat; only exercise does that job. Some foods with caffeine may speed up your metabolism (the way your body uses calories) for a short time, but they don't cause weight loss.

Myth: Natural or herbal weight-loss products are safe and effective.

Fact: A weight-loss product that claims to be "natural" or "herbal" is not necessarily safe. These products are not usually scientifically tested to prove their effectiveness or safety. In the worst-case scenario they can even be harmful. For example, herbal products containing ephedra (now banned by the federal government) have caused serious health problems and even death. Newer products that claim to be ephedra-free are not necessarily danger-free, because they may contain ingredients similar to ephedra.

Myth: Skipping meals is a good way to lose weight.

Fact: Studies show that people who skip breakfast and eat fewer times during the day tend to be heavier than people who eat a healthy breakfast and eat four or five small meals a day. This may be because people who skip meals tend to feel hungrier later on, and eat more than they normally would. It may also be that eating many small meals throughout the day helps people control their appetites. If you take diabetes medication to control blood glucose, you are at risk of low blood sugar when you skip meals.

Myth: Eating after 8 p.m. causes weight gain.

Fact: It doesn't matter what time of day you eat. It is what and how much you eat and how much physical activity you do during the whole day that determines whether you gain, lose, or maintain your weight. No matter when you eat, your body will store extra calories as fat.

Power Points

☞ Weight loss is one of the best ways to manage your diabetes.

☞ Two common reasons for being overweight are eating too much and not being active enough.

☞ Abdominal fat is associated with a greater risk for heart disease and insulin resistance.

☞ A healthy body mass index (BMI) is less than 25.

☞ Waist measurements more than 40 inches for men and 35 inches for women are indicators of increased risk for heart disease and high blood pressure.

☞ A slow gradual weight loss of one half to one pound weekly is best.

☞ Discuss your weight loss goals with your diabetes dream team.

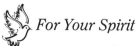 *For Your Spirit*

What Are You Willing to Give Up?

Oh, how their feet must have ached. Back in the day, folks worked on the farm, in the mill, in other folk's houses cooking and cleaning and chasing after children—on their feet all day. Of course their feet were tired—too tired to walk home after an all-day shift. But if the folks in Montgomery had to walk, they did. To have ridden a bus during the bus boycotts would have been an act of betrayal. It was a personal sacrifice to walk or wait for an uncertain ride, but people understood that it was important to their community. They may *not* have known how their singular act, in a small city in Alabama, would gain national attention and become a defining moment in American history.

That is the way with sacrifice. What you forfeit may be a small thing, a temporary inconvenience—but you have no idea how far reaching the benefits of your sacrifice may be.

It can be hard to remember that when you're being asked to give up something you want or something you are accustomed to doing. If you can't move your thinking beyond what you want today—*right now*—you'll only balk at the trouble and inconvenience of not being able to do what you want to do. The task is to remind yourself that what feels good or tastes good or sounds good right now, may not be the thing that will sustain you into the future.

That's certainly the case with diet, isn't it? *Oh, I'll just have a little cake,* we think. We eat it and it's gone. But its effects linger—on our hips, in our blood sugar—affecting our health and reminding us later of the sacrifice we *didn't* make. That's why your diabetes dream team keeps reminding you of the complications that can arise if you don't take good care of your condition. Taking the time to check your feet now can help you avoid an amputation later. Controlling your blood sugar carefully may mean you avoid dialysis in the future.

Sacrifice is an act of faith—that the thing you forfeit now will be a small price to pay for the reward you will receive later. It is like a tiny seed planted in the ground; you have no idea how large it will grow or what great fruit it will bear. But if you walk in faith, the way the citizens of Montgomery did, you can rest assured that your sacrifice will be rewarded.

12 GET A MOVE ON: EXERCISING TO CONTROL DIABETES

Food, food, food! People with diabetes hear about diet, nutrition and meal plans all the time. What you eat and how you eat is vitally important to controlling diabetes. But you should know that exercise is just as beneficial as diet for people with diabetes.

If you are like many people, the word "exercise" brings back memories of the hundreds of jumping jacks, pushups, laps and other calisthenics that you were forced to do in school. Those sweaty classes were often among the most dreaded. But when you were out playing stickball with your friends or shooting hoops or speeding down the street on your bike you were having fun. The word exercise never crossed your mind—but that's exactly what you were doing.

Exercise is actually any physical activity that gets your body moving above a resting level. It doesn't need to have a structured or formal plan; you can make it a part of your everyday routine—walking to the bus stop, dancing at a party on the weekend, cutting the grass, or chasing your grandchildren.

The key to fitting in exercise is to make it something enjoyable and fun—something you're going to look forward to doing. If you carefully choose activities that fit your schedule and your temperament, you might be surprised at how easy it is to add it to your diabetes management. You can do it.

Why Do It?

Why is exercise as important as diet in diabetes management? The list goes on and on. It can lower your blood glucose, blood pressure, and bad cholesterol, while increasing your good cholesterol. It improves your body's ability to use insulin, which might allow you to decrease the amount of medication you need. It lowers your risk of heart disease and stroke—both of which are disease risks among people with diabetes. It keeps your heart and bones strong and your joints flexible. You will have more energy, less stress, and a clearer mind. And, if you work it right, you may lose weight and body fat as well.

We also know that, if you have pre-diabetes, exercise can actually prevent the onset of type 2 diabetes.

What Activities Should You Include to Get All These Benefits?

There are four categories of exercise—aerobic exercise, strength training, stretching, and being extra active every day. You should try to get a little of each into your weekly exercise plan.

Let's look at that last one first because this is the easiest to start with. Being **extra active** every day is a simple matter of moving more as you go about your daily tasks. Walk instead of drive, take the stairs instead of the elevator, park further away from the store, or walk the kids home from school; on the weekends when you have more time, spend an hour tending your garden. Even vacuuming your house more often can help—pushing and pulling that heavy machine can help you work up a sweat. (Clean rugs are just a bonus.) Add 15 minutes of activity to your daily routine and gradually work your way up to 30 minutes. A little extra movement will help you burn more calories daily.

Aerobic exercise is exercise that increases your heart rate and your rate of breathing. When you exercise aerobically your body uses oxygen as it breaks down fat and glucose for energy. This type of exercise requires you to move the large muscles, which boost the heart rate. Formal aerobic exercise is designed or supervised by a professional and includes aerobic videotapes, riding a stationary bike, running or walking on a treadmill, taking an aerobics or water aerobics class or using a stair climber. Informal aerobic exercise includes walking briskly, hiking, climbing stairs, swimming, playing tennis, cross-country skiing, inline skating, ice-skating, riding a bicycle, or dancing.

Exercise experts recommend that you do 30 minutes of moderate-intensity aerobic exercise each day, most days of the week. The intensity of exercise is a measure of how hard your body is working and the "talk test" is an easy way to judge your activity level. Light intensity activities should allow you to sing while you're doing them. You should be able to belt out your Aretha Franklin favorites while you walk on the treadmill. If you are aiming for moderate intensity activity such as walking briskly, you should be able to carry on a conversation without huffing and puffing while walking. You're exercising vigorously if you are too winded or out of breath to carry on a conversation. But if you haven't been physically active for a while, you should start with light activity and work your way up to at least a moderate level.

▶ Light intensity activities include walking slowly, golfing using a powered cart, swimming slowly, gardening or pruning, bicycling with very little effort, dusting, vacuuming, or light stretching.

▶ Moderate intensity activities include walking briskly, golfing pulling or carrying your own clubs, recreational swimming, using a power mower to mow the lawn, playing doubles tennis, bicycling 5 to 9 mph, scrubbing floors or washing windows, or weight lifting.

▶ Vigorous intensity activities include race walking, jogging or running, swimming laps, mowing the lawn with a hand mower, playing singles tennis, bicycling more than 10 mph, moving furniture, or circuit training.

If you can't carve out 30 minutes daily for your physical activities there is no need to worry. You can break it up into three 10 minute segments, or two 15 segments. Get it in where you can fit it in.

Strength training, sometimes known as weight lifting or resistance training, helps you build strong bones and muscles. There are many good reasons to include strength training as part of your physical activities.

▶ Increase muscle strength and flexibility.

▶ Decrease insulin resistance leading to improved glucose control.

▶ Increase metabolism allowing you to burn more calories daily.

▶ Build and maintain bone density.

▶ Reduce pain and stiffness associated with arthritis.

▶ Reduce heart disease risk.

▶ Strengthen back and abdominal muscles.

▶ Improve balance and coordination.

▶ Improve appearance.

Strength training when done in combination with aerobic exercise can also improve your mental and emotional health.

Experts recommend that you do strength training two to three times a week. You can make it part of your 30 minutes of moderate-intensity physical activity each day. If you can't get to a gym to use weight machines, you can do weight workouts at home with dumbbells, elastic exercise bands, weighted balls, or even using your own body weight as resistance.

Your diabetes dream team can tell you more about what kind of strength training is best for you. Having a personal trainer may also be helpful if you haven't done strength training before, but be sure that the trainer has a degree in exercise physiology or is certified through the American College of Sports Medicine—and tell him or her you have diabetes.

Stretching is the last category of exercise, but not the least. Stretching increases muscle and joint flexibility and range of motion so you can move your joins and limbs fully. It keeps you from being sore after exercise, relieves stress, and makes it easier to perform daily activities like bending down to tie your shoes. Some formal types of exercises that focus on flexibility include yoga, tai chi, and Pilates, but you can find simple ways to fit stretching into your daily routine. Touch your toes ten times before you get out of bed, really reach for the items on the top shelf of the cabinet, lunge into each stroke with the mop.

Stretch slowly—don't bounce—and hold the stretch for 30 seconds. Breathe normally; don't hold your breath. If you haven't stretched before, you may only be able to hold the stretch for a few seconds. Your goal is to work your way up until you can hold each stretch for 30 seconds. Although stretching sounds easy enough, there may be stretches that you should not do. For example, if you have a back injury, stretching your back may be harmful.

The Mental Workout

If you have never exercised or it has been a long time since you last worked out, you need to know a few more things to keep you healthy and safe.

See your doctor before you start an exercise program. She will check you over to make sure it's safe for you to exercise. You may be asked to take a stress test—a test that tells the doctor how your heart reacts to exercise. Your doctor will also give you information specific to your condition. For instance, if you have retinopathy, eye damage from diabetes (more on this soon), you may be told to avoid exercises like weight lifting as this can cause further damage to the eye.

Once your doc gives you the go ahead to exercise, you will need to get yourself started.

Make detailed plans. Note the activities you plan to do and how you will do them. Make sure you choose activities that are realistic for you; they should be challenging but not too difficult. Remember to choose things you enjoy. The more you like an activity the more likely you are to do it daily. Remember to start slowly and to be flexible in your schedule. For instance, if it is extremely hot or cold out you might not want to workout outside. Have a backup plan: walk the mall or around an indoor track.

If you have a hard time starting a program, consider recruiting a friend to join you—it is always easier to stick to a program when you are with someone. You will be accountable to each other for getting up and out to exercise. Better yet, join or create a group of exercise buddies. If you partner with more than one person, if someone drops out, there will be others to keep the momentum going.

Reward yourself for meeting your goals for the week—but don't treat yourself with food. A manicure, a massage, or a movie night are good choices. Use the exercise worksheet at the end of this chapter to set your short-term goals, describe your plan, document your progress, and keep track of your planned rewards. It can be very motivating to track your progress and see how far you have come.

If you're not used to exercising, you will need to find some motivation to keep going. Sometimes just seeing the benefits can keep you moving, but six-pack abs or a ten-pound weight loss are benefits that take time to achieve. One way to see the benefits of exercise right away is to test your blood glucose before and after exercise. You'll be amazed at how exercise can help lower your glucose levels.

Checking your blood sugar is important for another reason as well. Exercise helps your body better use insulin, so if your blood sugar is high, exercise is a good thing. But if you're not careful you may experience hypoglycemia (low blood glucose) after you exercise. It's important for you to check your blood glucose before and after exercising; it may be necessary for you to test during exercise as well. If you find that your blood glucose is too low or too high before you exercise, you should wait until your glucose has recovered.

Checking your glucose before you exercise will help you decide whether you need a snack that can provide some additional glucose for fuel and to prevent hypoglycemia. If your blood glucose is below 100 mg/dL you should have a small snack. If you take insulin, ask your health-care team whether you should change your dosage before you exercise. Keeping a record of your blood glucose readings and exercise will help you develop your own individual exercise and snack guidelines. The following chart can serve as a general guideline to get you started.

Physical Activity and Snack Guidelines

Intensity	Duration (minutes)	Snack (Carbohydrate grams)	Frequency
Mild to moderate Walking slowly (1–2 mph) Bowling or vacuuming	30	May not be needed	———
Moderate Walking briskly (3 ½ mph) Hiking or dancing	30 to 60	15 grams 8 animal crackers or 1 medium piece of fruit	Each hour
High Running, jogging, Aerobics or chopping wood	60+	30 to 50 grams 8 animal crackers plus 1 cup milk or 1 turkey sandwich plus 1 cup milk	Each hour

If you're exercising and start to feel faint, dizzy, weak, confused, shaky, or nervous, or if you feel hungry, have a change in heart rate, or suddenly break out in extra sweat, you may be having a hypoglycemic episode. Check your blood glucose immediately. If it's below 70, take one of the following right away; 2 to 3 glucose tablets, 1/2 cup of fruit juice, 1/2 cup regular soda, 1 cup skim milk, 5 or 6 pieces of hard candy or a tablespoon or two of sugar or honey. Recheck your blood glucose after 15 minutes. If it's still less than 70 take another serving of sugar and repeat these steps until your blood glucose is at least 70.

If your blood glucose is over 300—or over 250 and you have ketones in your urine—don't exercise until your blood glucose drops. Test your ketone levels with a home urine test designed for that purpose. When they're back to normal *and* your blood glucose is below 250, it's safe to work out again.

Just as everyone has individual responses to diet and medication, everyone has an individual response to exercise. When it comes to exercise, you need to understand how exercise affects your blood glucose. You will be better able to prevent hypoglycemia or very high blood glucose if you know how you will respond to the exercise you have planned.

Treating Hypoglycemia

If your blood glucose is 70 or lower, have one of the following right away:

2 or 3 glucose tablets

1/2 cup (4 ounces) of any fruit juice

1/2 cup (4 ounces) of a regular (not diet) soft drink

1 cup (8 ounces) of skim milk

5 or 6 pieces of hard candy

1 or 2 tablespoons of sugar or honey

After 15 minutes, check your blood glucose again. If it's still too low, have another serving. Repeat until your blood glucose is 70 or higher. If it will be an hour or more before your next meal, have a snack as well.

Taking Care

When you work out you should always wear a diabetes identification bracelet or tag—which you should wear all the time anyway, just in case you lose consciousness from a hypoglycemic episode. You will want anyone who stops to help you to know that you have diabetes.

As you care for your diabetes, it is important to keep an eye on the health of your feet. If you are diabetic, simple injuries to your feet can turn into serious infections. Everyone with diabetes needs to check their feet daily, but if you are exercising you need to be especially careful. Always examine your feet before and after exercise, checking to make sure you don't have any sores or blisters. Wear smooth-fitting polyester or poly-blend socks that are soft and absorbent, and shoes that fit well, are comfortable and designed for the activity you are doing—walking shoes for walking, tennis shoes for tennis. Using a gel insert in your footwear might reduce your risk of blisters or sores. If you already suffer with poor circulation and/or have nerve damage in your feet, there may be some activities that you should skip. Choose an activity that doesn't put pressure on the feet, like swimming, yoga, tai chi, bicycling, rowing, chair exercises, or upper-body workouts.

Water is essential during exercise. It is important for you to drink plenty of sugar free liquids before, during, and after physical activity—especially when you exercise in hot conditions. Dehydration, not having enough water in your body, can increase your blood glucose. Having six to eight glasses of sugar-free fluid a day should keep you well hydrated, unless you're exercising extremely vigorously; then you might need more.

One last important precaution: If you use insulin you need to be careful where you inject it. You should inject it in your abdomen, not your arm or leg muscles. Because those muscles are working hard during exercise, the insulin that you injected will be absorbed much faster. This can result in a hypoglycemic reaction.

Power Points

☞ Physical activity can lower your blood glucose, blood pressure, and bad cholesterol.

☞ You should aim for 30 minutes of physical activity daily.

☞ Aerobic exercise, strength training, stretching, and being extra active are all part of physical activity. You should try to get a little of each every day.

☞ Check with your doctor before you start an exercise program.

☞ Be sure your wear diabetes identification.

☞ Always carry glucose tablets, hard candy, or juice when exercising in case you have a hypoglycemic reaction—low blood sugar.

☞ If exercising alone, tell someone where you will be exercising.

☞ Drink plenty of sugar-free liquids before, during, and after exercise.

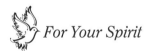 *For Your Spirit*

Putting the Disciple Back in Discipline

Talk to any athletic coach and he'll tell you the secret to winning is discipline—discipline in practice, discipline in play. When you hear the word discipline you may think of punishment—spare the rod, spoil the child. Or, in the context of fitness, you may think of the no-pain, no-gain boot-camp approach that says you push yourself to your maximum. If you're stiff with pain tomorrow, you'll know you were doing it right. *Now drop and give me 50.*

But the origin of the word *discipline* is the same as *disciple*. It means pupil—someone who studies and follows instruction. Discipline actually means behaving in a controlled, orderly way. It's not working harder, it's about working smarter—following the wisest path.

When you decide that you want to eat better, lose weight, get fit, or do anything that's good for you, instead of launching into a hard-core regimen of deprivation and overwork, create a program that you can manage and sustain in the long-term. If you start out working out too hard or too intensely, it will be harder for you to keep up the pace over time.

This is your life—not a temporary fitness program, that you can go at hard and go home. You need to find a program that can become a part of the order of your life. Be gentle with yourself, making reasonable fitness goals and striving to meet them without beating yourself up. Yes, you have to work at it—you have to feel the exertion, you have to motivate yourself to keep at it. But in the end the discipline is in learning what to do and following your own good wisdom.

Sample Exercise Worksheet

Week of: March 19th	Goal for week: walk 3x, yoga 1x, weights 2x		Reward for meeting goal of the week: go to movies with Mary on Saturday				
	PLAN		ACTUAL				
Day/date	Exercise Type (A = aerobic, S = strength, F = flexibility) Exercise (where, how, with what, etc.)	Time	Blood sugar before	Feet: Before & After	Exercise	Time Spent	Blood sugar after
Monday 3/19	A - Walk fitness trail at beach during lunch break	30 Min	110	☐ ☐	Walk at mall - rain	25 min	90
Tuesday 3/20	S - Lift weights at home using Donna Richardson tape	20 Min	130	☐ ☐	Lifted weights	20 min	101
Wednesday	A – walk with Mary at the park after work	30 Min					
Thursday	F – Yoga class at the gym after work	60 Min					
Friday	S - Lift weights at home using Donna Richardson tape	20 Min					
Saturday	A – walk with Bill around town	40 Min					
Sunday	Walk to church/ walk home after service	30 Min					
		Total					

Notes (list any extra daily activities, problems, or questions):
Parked at other end of parking lot at mall allowing me to walk further before and after exercise.

Exercise Worksheet

Week of:	Goal for week:				Reward for meeting goal of the week:		
	PLAN			ACTUAL			
Day/date	Exercise Type (A = aerobic, S = strength, F = flexibility) Exercise (where, how, with what, etc.)	Time	Blood sugar before	Feet: Before & After	Exercise	Time Spent	Blood sugar after

Notes (list any extra daily activities, problems, or questions):

13 TAKE THAT!
MEDICATIONS AND TREATMENTS

No one includes a diabetes diagnosis in their hopes and dreams for the future. However, if you're diagnosed with diabetes in the 21st century, there is good news: we know how to successfully treat and manage diabetes.

Diet, exercise, and SMBG are always at the forefront of diabetes management. But when diet and exercise alone are not enough to keep your glucose at safe levels, it's comforting to know effective medications are available. Since diabetes was identified as a disease, researchers have discovered a variety of oral medications, insulin, and other injectables to effectively manage diabetes.

You might be surprised to know that 9 out of every 10 people with diabetes require diabetes medications, insulin injections, or both to reach the glucose targets. And though people don't like the idea of taking medicine—especially something you have to take every day for the rest of your life, it's important to remember that keeping your blood glucose levels as close to normal as possible can prevent or slow the progression of serious diabetes complications. Medication can be the key to keeping that from happening.

Diabetes Medication Myths

People tend to be confused about diabetes medicines because there are so many of them, the science and technology of delivering them has changed over time, and different people need different meds depending on their condition. Aunt Julie's diabetes may be different from Uncle Leo's, so their medicine regimen may be as well. The result is that there a lot of myths about the medicine.

Myth: Once you start taking diabetes medicine you can never stop.

Fact: There are temporary conditions such as surgery that cause elevated glucose levels and require insulin. But after surgery, with continued emphasis on healthy eating habits and regular physical activity, glucose levels may be controlled without medication.

Myth: If you don't take diabetes medicine your diabetes must not be serious.

Fact: Not everyone who has diabetes takes diabetes medicine. If the body produces some insulin, then weight loss, healthy eating habits, and regular physical activity can help insulin work more effectively. However, diabetes does change over time, and diabetes medicine may be needed later.

Myth: Once you start taking diabetes medicine you can eat anything you want.

Fact: Your diabetes medicine is more effective when you follow a healthy eating plan. And when you're eating healthy you might not need as much medicine to lower your blood glucose levels.

Myth: Insulin pills can help control diabetes.

Fact: Insulin is a protein; it cannot be taken by mouth because it would be digested by the stomach. Insulin must be given by injection or through an insulin pump in the skin. There are pills for diabetes that help by making the body produce more insulin, use its own insulin better, produce less blood glucose from the liver, or limit carbohydrate absorption after a meal.

Myth: If I need insulin, it means I failed to manage my diabetes.

Fact: Most people with type 2 diabetes will eventually need to use insulin because diabetes is a progressive disease that changes through time. If diabetes pills no longer keep your blood glucose levels in a safe range, it is not because you failed at taking care of yourself.

Myth: Insulin is a cure for diabetes.

Fact: Insulin is not a cure for diabetes. There is no cure—at least not yet. There are only medicine and behaviors that can control diabetes. Insulin helps do that by keeping the blood glucose from rising.

Let's take a look at the oral medications, insulin and other injectable medicine—by category, brand name and generic name. (It is important to learn both names.) The generic name will be listed first, followed by the brand names.

Oral Agents

In the 1950s, a pharmacologist testing sulfonylurea as a treatment for typhoid found that it lowered blood sugar. His discovery led to the first oral anti-diabetic drug for use in people with type 2 diabetes. There are now six classes of oral diabetes medications, each class working in a unique way to control your glucose levels. These medications help the body produce more insulin, use its own insulin better, produce less glucose from the liver, or limit carbohydrate absorption after a meal.

Sulfonylureas

This class of medications lowers blood glucose levels by stimulating the cells that produce insulin (beta cells) in the pancreas. Sulfonylureas have the greatest impact on your fasting glucose levels. Some of the side effects that can be seen with this class of medications include hypoglycemia (low blood glucose), stomach upset, skin rash, itching, hives, rash, sun sensitivity, and weight gain. You should not take sulfonylureas if you are pregnant, have serious liver or kidney disease, or you are allergic to sulfa drugs.

> ▷ Glipizide (Glucotrol). This medication, approved in 1984, is usually taken once daily, on an empty stomach, 30 minutes before breakfast, in a dose of 5–40 mg daily. However, some people do better with 2 or 3 smaller doses throughout the day. Your doctor will discuss these options with you. It is also available in an extended release tablet called Glucotrol XL at a maximum dose of 20 mg. Glucotrol XL should only be given once daily with breakfast.

> ▷ Glyburide (Diabeta, Glycron, Glynase, Micronase). This medication is usually taken once a day with the first main meal, in a dose range of 1.25–20 mg daily. Again, this medication might work better if it is given in smaller doses twice a day, but your doctor will discuss this with you if this is the drug of choice.

> ▷ Glimepiride (Amaryl). This medication is administered as a single dose taken in the morning with breakfast, in a dose that you take is based on your individual response to this medication.

Meglitinides

This class of medication is also called non-sulfonylurea secretagogues, because they trigger the release of insulin from the pancreas just like sulfonylureas, but they will only trigger the release of insulin if blood sugar is elevated, which reduces the chances that you will suffer from hypoglycemia (low blood sugar). Side effects include diarrhea, dizziness, headache, hypoglycemia, and weight gain. Meglitinides are most effective on after-meal glucose levels.

▷ Nateglinide (Starlix). The medication is usually taken 1 to 30 minutes before meals, 2 to 4 times a day. The dose range is 180 mg to 360 mg daily.

▷ Repaglinide (Prandin). This is usually taken three times a day within 15 minutes of each meal. Don't take it if you skip a meal. The dose range is 1.5 mg to 16 mg daily.

Thiazolidinediones

This class of medication, also known as glitazones or TZDs, lowers blood glucose by making cells more sensitive to insulin, which decreases insulin resistance—helping glucose enter the cells more easily. It also reduces the amount of stored glucose your liver releases. Because of its action on the liver, your doctor will probably want to check your liver function before he prescribes it. If you have congestive heart failure or liver disease you can't take a TZD at all. It has side effects that might include liver failure, respiratory infection, headache, fluid retention, and weight gain. This medication takes several weeks to work and may therefore take some time before your correct dose is finally determined.

▷ Pioglitazone (Actos). You take 15–45 mg of this one once daily—and you won't have to worry about taking this medication with or before meals.

▷ Rosiglitazone (Avandia). This medication is usually taken in either one dose in the morning or a divided dose twice a day. The dose range is 4–8 mg daily. Don't worry about taking it with meals or before meals.

Biguanide

This class of medication lowers your blood sugar by improving insulin's ability to move glucose into cells, particularly muscle cells. It also prevents your liver from releasing its stored glucose, decreases the amount of glucose absorbed in the intestines, and can possibly cause a modest weight loss. Biguanides have the greatest impact on your fasting blood glucose levels.

If you have kidney damage, liver damage, or heart failure, this isn't the medicine for you. Side effects include diarrhea, nausea, abdominal bloating, cramping, loss of appetite, and a metallic taste in the mouth. If you are taking a biguanide, remind your doctor. You may have to stop taking the medication for a few days if you need surgery or tests that require a dye.

▷ Metformin (Glucophage). A dose of 500 to 2500 mg daily of standard metformin can be taken either 2 or 3 times a day with meals to prevent stomach upset. In 2000, the FDA approved Glucophage XR, an extended release version of metformin. This medication is long-lasting, so it only needs to be taken once a day with dinner. The dose range is 500 mg to 1000 mg daily.

If you have difficulty swallowing tablets, metformin is also available as a liquid called Riomet. A 5 ml dose is equivalent to 500 mg metformin.

Alpha-Glucosidase Inhibitors

This class of medication is very different than all the others mentioned because it works by blocking the absorption of glucose in the intestines. This slows down the rise in blood glucose that occurs with starch intake. Alpha-Glucosidase Inhibitors have the greatest impact on your after-meal blood glucose levels. The most common side effects of alpha-glucosidase inhibitors are upset stomach, including gas, diarrhea, nausea, and cramps. Because of the way the drugs work in the intestines, you can't take alpha-glucosidase inhibitors if you have chronic intestinal disease.

> ▸ Acarbose (Precose). Acarbose should be taken with the first bite of each of your main meals—usually three times a day in a 75 to 300 mg dose.

> ▸ Miglitol (Glyset). This medication is taken the same way Acarbose: 75–300 mg three times a day with the first bite of a meal.

Dipeptidyl Peptidase-4 (DPP-4) Inhibitor

This is a new class of medication, also known as gliptins, first approved by the FDA in late 2006. This new class works by stopping the body from turning off GLP-1, a gut hormone that causes your body to release insulin in response to elevated glucose levels after a meal. By making GLP-1 stay active, gliptins help the body continue to release insulin. At the same time, it prevents your liver from making glucose, which also lowers you blood glucose levels. Because gliptins are glucose dependent they don't cause hypoglycemia. Side effects of gliptins are upper respiratory infection, headache, and diarrhea.

> ▸ Sitagliptin phosphate (Januvia). This medication is taken once a day in a 25 to 100 mg dose.

> ▸ Saxagliptin (Onglyza). FDA approved in July 2009, saxagliptin is taken once a day without regard to meals. Dose range is 2.5mg to 5 mg.

Fixed Combinations

This is not really a true medication class, because it combines meds from each of the classes. Because the previously mentioned oral medications all work in different ways, some of the medications that are used to treat type 2 diabetes are combined with others, all in one pill. The following lists of medications are combinations of the medications we just reviewed.

▸ Glipizide/Metformin (Metaglip). This medication is taken once or twice a day at a dose of 2.5/250 mg to 5/500 mg. When taking this medication, you must drink plenty of fluids. It can take up to two weeks for you to see the full benefit of this medication.

▸ Glyburide/Metformin (Glucovance). This medication is taken one or two times a day with meals. Like Metaglip, it takes a couple of weeks to work and you must drink plenty of fluids while taking this medication. The dose range is 1.25mg/250 mg to 5mg/500 mg.

▸ Pioglitazone/Glimepiride (Duetact). This is usually taken once a day with your first main meal. The dose range is 30mg/2 mg to 30mg/4mg.

▸ Pioglitazone/Metformin (Actoplus Met). It is usually taken once or twice daily with a meal. The dose range is 15mg/500mg to 15mg/850mg.

▸ Rosiglitazone/Glimepiride (Avandaryl). This medication is only taken with the first meal of the day, but it may take 2 to 3 months for the drug to fully take effect. The dose range is 4mg/1mg to 8mg/4mg.

▸ Rosiglitazone/Metformin (Avandamet). It is taken once or twice a day with food in a 2mg/500mg to 4mg/1000mg dose

▸ Sitagliptin/Metformin (Janumet). It is taken twice daily with meals. The dose range is 50 mg/500 mg to 100 mg/2000 mg.

It's important to keep track of what kind of oral diabetes medicine you take. Use the form at the end of this chapter to write down the names of your diabetes medicine, the amount you take, how often, and when you take them. Take this record with you when visiting any member of your diabetes dream team or any other medical professional who treats you.

Non-Insulin Injectables

These medications belong to a class known as incretin mimetics, which mimic the actions of the natural hormones in the body that stimulate the pancreas to secrete insulin. Because they are hormones, these medications need to be injected; biological and synthetic hormones are proteins that would be digested in your stomach if you took them orally so they won't work the way they should. Because incretin mimetics are glucose dependent, they will only cause your body to release insulin in response to elevated glucose levels after a meal. This lowers the risk of hypoglycemia. They also prevent your liver from making glucose, which also lowers your blood glucose levels. Incretin mimetics may help you lose a little weight, too, because they slow the rate that food leaves the stomach, which helps you feel satisfied with less food. Side effects are diarrhea, nausea, and vomiting. There are currently two drugs in this class.

⬧ Exenatide (Byetta). This medication works by acting like the GLP-1 hormone, which causes your body to release insulin in the response to high sugar levels after a meal. It's injected under the skin in the thigh, abdomen, or upper arm two times a day within the hour before breakfast and dinner. Dose range is 5 mcg to 20 mcg.

⬧ Pramlintide Acetate (Symlin). The medication works by acting like the hormone amylin. This hormone works to control your blood sugar by slowing the movement of food through the stomach. At the same time it decreases your appetite and the amount of sugar your liver makes. This medication is injected into either the stomach or thigh before each major meal. A major meal is one that contains at least 250 calories or at least 30 g of carbohydrates. Dose range is 15 mcg to 120 mcg.

Insulin

Insulin has come a long, long way since the first doctors used it to treat diabetes. In the early years of insulin use, insulin was taken from animals such as the cow or pig. When we learned how to manufacturer a synthetic form of human insulin that is identical to the insulin our pancreas makes, the man-made form replaced animal forms of the hormone. In fact, as of January 2006, animal hormones were no longer approved for production or sale in the United States.

Science has advanced to a point that we can adjust the insulin molecule, creating modified insulin preparations called insulin analogs. This new insulin differs slightly from the original insulin and, in turn, changes how quickly the insulin will work.

Insulin products are available in four basic forms. These forms have a different time of onset (how soon it starts to work), peak (when it works the hardest), and duration (how long it lasts in the body). These features are the major factors your doctor considers in choosing the right insulin for you.

People with type 1 diabetes need daily insulin injections to live, but people with type 2 only got it as a last resort. However recent research has led to a paradigm shift; insulin therapy is now initiated much earlier in the course of type 2. Many people with type 2 diabetes are treated with insulin in combination with oral medications. Early initiation of basal insulin helps to improve fasting glucose levels, so the oral agents tend to work better. People who are unable to achieve appropriate hormone levels despite maximal doses of oral medications are prime candidates for insulin therapy.

▶ Rapid Acting insulin products generally start working rapidly but don't last very long.

　▷ Insulin Aspart (Novolog) starts working in about 10 to 20 minutes, peaks at about 1 to 3 hours, and finishes working in about 3 to 4 hours.

　▷ Insulin Glulisine (Apidra) starts working about 15 to 20 minutes, peaks about 1 hour, and lasts about 5 hours.

　▷ Insulin Lispro (Humalog) starts working 5 to 15 minutes, peaks at about 45 to 90 minutes, and lasts 3 to 4 hours.

▶ Short Acting insulin products generally take a little longer to start working and work for a short period of time.

　▷ Insulin Regular Human (Humulin R and Novolin R) starts working in about 30 minutes, peaking at 2 to 5 hours, and stops working at 5 to 8 hours.

▶ Intermediate Acting insulin preparations take longer to start working but last much longer than the rapid or short acting insulin products.

　▷ Insulin Human Isophane also known as NPH insulin (Humulin N and Novolin N). This intermediate acting insulin starts working about 1 to 3 hours, peaks at 6 to 12 hours, and finishes its job between 16 to 24 hours.

▶ Long Acting insulin products take a long time to start working but work for a very long time.

　▷ Insulin Detemir (Levemir) has a "peakless" action, which means that it works evenly through its duration—which is between 6 and 24 hours. This large variation depends on dose and other factors related to your individual diagnosis.

⊳ Insulin Glargine (Lantus) also has a "peakless" action, evenly working between 11 to more than 24 hours.

Pre-mixed Insulin

The insulin in your body works in a very precise way: insulin levels normally vary throughout the day based on your blood glucose levels. Picture a roller coaster and you have an idea of what your daily insulin levels look like. A small amount of insulin that floats around our blood stream all the time—*basal insulin*. After meals when our blood glucose rises, insulin increases to bring the glucose back down to "normal." These peaks of insulin are called *bolus insulin*. Basal insulin is best mimicked using intermediate- and long-acting insulin preparations, while bolus insulin is best mimicked using rapid-acting or short-acting insulin products. Instead of having to take three or four injections of insulin a day to cover all the insulin needs, using pre-mixed insulin cuts that down to two or three injections a day because it has a mixture of these insulin products.

⊳ Insulin Aspart Protamine/Insulin Aspart (NovoLog Mix 70/30). This insulin pre-mix is 70 percent intermediate acting and 30 percent rapid acting insulin. It starts working faster and lasts longer than regular insulin alone.

⊳ Insulin Lispro Protamine/Insulin Lispro (Humalog Mix). This insulin pre-mix is 75 percent intermediate acting insulin and 25 percent rapid acting insulin. It starts working faster and lasts longer than regular insulin alone.

⊳ Insulin Human Isophane Suspension 50/Regular 50 (Novolin 50/50). Half intermediate acting insulin and half short acting insulin, it starts to work as quickly as regular insulin but lasts longer.

⊳ Insulin Human Isophane Suspension 70/Regular 30 (Novolin 70/30). This insulin mix is 70 percent intermediate acting insulin and 30 percent short-acting insulin. It also works quickly and lasts longer.

Prescription Assistance

During the past 23 years, advances in diabetes medicines and treatment have sky rocketed. At the same time, the cost of health insurance and prescription drug coverage has increased. Employers are contributing less and requiring employees to pay more for medical benefits. Often people will opt for health plans that do not have adequate prescription coverage or no coverage because they are less expensive.

When you have diabetes it is important that you have health insurance that will support your needs. Regular contact with your diabetes dream team and taking your medication as prescribed are the keys to living healthy with diabetes. If you can't afford prescription drug coverage, you may be eligible for prescription assistance.

Most pharmaceutical companies offer prescription assistance to people who are uninsured or underinsured. Many of these companies belong to a nationwide program known as the Partnership for Prescription Assistance (PPA). The mission of the PPA is to increase awareness of the many patient assistance programs available and boost enrollment of those who are eligible.

If you need prescription assistance, call the PPA at 1-888-4PPA-NOW (1-888-477-2669) or visit them online at *www.PPARX.org.* You will be matched with the program that's right for you. Your medication will be provided free or nearly free.

Taking your diabetes medication as prescribed is an important part of successful diabetes management. Your diabetes dream team can also assist you in getting the medications that you need.

Power Points

☞ Most people with diabetes require diabetes medicine, insulin injections, or both to reach blood glucose targets.

☞ Keeping your blood glucose in the target range can prevent or slow down the progression of diabetes complications.

☞ Oral diabetes medicines help your body produce more insulin, use its' own insulin better, produce less blood glucose from the liver, or limit carbohydrate absorption.

☞ You should know the generic and brand name of your diabetes medicine.

☞ Diabetes medicine is more effective when you follow a healthy eating plan.

☞ Insulin is not a cure for diabetes; it helps to control diabetes by keeping your blood glucose from rising.

☞ If you can't afford your diabetes medicines contact the Partnership for Prescription Assistance, 1-888-477-2669 or *www.PPARX.org.*

My Diabetes Medicines
(Sample)

Fill in the names of your diabetes medicines. Look at the box "What Diabetes Medicines Can Do" and find your diabetes medicines class. Then write down the class, generic and brand name, the amount to take, how often, and when to take. Do this for all your diabetes medicines. Your doctor or any member of your diabetes dream team can help you fill in this record. It is a good idea to write this in pencil so you can easily make changes when your doctor makes changes in your diabetes medicines.

Class of Medicine: *Biguanides*

Generic Name: *Metformin*

Brand Name: *Glucophage*

Amount: *500mg* How Often: *2x daily*

When to take: *With dinner*

Class of Medicine:_____

Generic Name:_____

Brand Name:_____

Amount:_____ How Often:_____

When to take:_____

Class of Medicine:_____

Generic Name:_____

Brand Name:_____

Amount:_____ How Often:_____

When to take:_____

Class of Medicine:_____

Generic Name:_____

Brand Name:_____

Amount:_____ How Often:_____

When to take:_____

What Diabetes Medicine Can Do

Alpha-glucosidase inhibitors
Slow down the rate at which glucose gets into your blood after eating.

Biguanides
Lower the amount of stored glucose released from the liver and helps glucose enter the cells.

Dipeptidyl peptidase-4 (DPP-4)
Helps incretin hormones stay active and stimulates the release of insulin. Also stops your liver from releasing stored glucose into your blood.

Meglitinides
Help your pancreas make more insulin.

Incretin Mimetics
Help your body release insulin in response to high blood sugar after meals. Keeps liver from releasing stored glucose.

Sulfonylureas
Help your body make more insulin.

Thiazolidinediones
Lower your insulin resistance and helps glucose enter the cells.

My Diabetes Medicines

Fill in the names of your diabetes medicines. Look at the box "What Diabetes Medicines Can Do" and find your diabetes medicines class. Then write down the class, generic and brand name, the amount to take, how often, and when to take. Do this for all your diabetes medicines. Your doctor or any member of your diabetes dream team can help you fill in this record. It is a good idea to write this in pencil so you can easily make changes when your doctor makes changes in your diabetes medicines.

Class of Medicine:_____

Generic Name:_____

Brand Name:_____

Amount:_____How Often:_____

When to take:_____

Class of Medicine:_____

Generic Name:_____

Brand Name:_____

Amount:_____How Often:_____

When to take:_____

Class of Medicine:_____

Generic Name:_____

Brand Name:_____

Amount:_____How Often:_____

When to take:_____

Class of Medicine:_____

Generic Name:_____

Brand Name:_____

Amount:_____How Often:_____

When to take:_____

What Diabetes Medicine Can Do

Alpha-glucosidase inhibitors
Slow down the rate at which glucose gets into your blood after eating.

Biguanides
Lower the amount of stored glucose released from the liver and helps glucose enter the cells.

Dipeptidyl peptidase-4 (DPP-4)
Helps incretin hormones stay active and stimulates the release of insulin. Also stops your liver from releasing stored glucose into your blood.

Meglitinides
Help your pancreas make more insulin.

Incretin Mimetics
Help your body release insulin in response to high blood sugar after meals. Keeps liver from releasing stored glucose.

Sulfonylureas
Help your body make more insulin.

Thiazolidinediones
Lower your insulin resistance and helps glucose enter the cells.

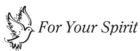 *For Your Spirit*

Faith in Things Unseen

The doctor rips the prescription off the pad and hands it to you. Later you hand it to the pharmacist and get a bottle of pills in return. You take them home, read the instructions, and swallow them down, just like the doctor ordered.

But you have no idea what you just took. What was in that pill? There's no nutrition information label on the bottle—just that page of all the scary side effects of the medication. Who knows what complex mix of chemicals and compounds were stirred together in a lab and made into the tablets you're taking. All you know is that the doctor said they would help. So you take them—your little tablets of faith. You don't know exactly how, but you believe they will help.

Hebrew says, "Now faith is the substance of things hoped for, the evidence of things not seen." You hope to stay well, whole, and healthy, and you turn to your doctor and the other members of the dream team to help you find your way to wellness. That's an act of faith. You trust that your care provider knows what he's talking about and is telling you what to do to ease your condition. (Or you should. If you don't, you're going to the wrong doctor.) You believe that the medication he gives you will work, so you take it and wait to see the evidence.

You don't ever know in advance how things are going to work. That particular prescription may not be potent enough; your insulin dose may need to change. And who knows what stage your condition will be in two months or two years or 10 years down the road. But you do what you believe, today, will keep you well tomorrow. That is faith in things unseen.

14 WHAT NEXT? AVOIDING DIABETES COMPLICATIONS

In the late 1800s, after a person was diagnosed with diabetes, he could expect to live, on average, only one to eight more years. With the discovery of insulin in the 1920s, people were able to live longer, but they still lived with debilitating complications of the disease. Over the years, as medicines and treatments improved, life expectancy has increased. It's higher now than it has ever been. Still, today the life expectancy for people with type 1 diabetes may be 15 years shorter than average. For those with type 2, life expectancy is reduced by 5 to 10 years.

As we learned more about diabetes, we learned that it was not so much diabetes itself that killed people; it was the complications. We know that, for the most part, complications occur from cell damage as a result of a persistent elevation of blood glucose. Treatment now focuses on keeping blood glucose down to avoid that cell damage and prevent complications—extending life and improving quality of life.

Your diabetes dream team will be working to help you avoid both short term (acute) complications, and those that occur in the long-term (chronic complications).

Acute Complications

Hypoglycemia

Hypoglycemia is also called low blood glucose or low blood sugar. You might be thinking, "I thought diabetes was high blood sugar, so how is low blood sugar a complication of diabetes?" It does seem strange, but consider this: diabetes causes high levels of glucose in the blood because the body's ability to balance glucose metabolism is not functioning as it should. Diabetes treatment is aimed at normalizing blood glucose and balancing glucose metabolism. But since you are balancing your glucose levels "artificially" with medicine, diet, and exercise—I often refer to this as shifting your own gears—there are times that your blood glucose might go too low.

If you're taking medications or insulin, hypoglycemia (blood sugar below 70) can occur as a result of skipped, delayed, or too-small meals; too much insulin or oral medications; increased amounts of exercise or activity; or excessive alcohol consumption. You may feel shaky, dizzy, sweaty, hungry, headache-y, clumsy, or confused. Someone may notice a change in your behavior. You could even have a seizure or pass out. Untreated, it can kill you.

If you start to experience any symptoms of hypoglycemia, check your blood glucose levels immediately. If your reading is less than 70, try to raise your blood glucose quickly by practicing "the rule of 15." Take 15 grams of carbs: 2 to 3 glucose tablets, 4 ounces of fruit juice, 4 ounces of regular soda, 1 cup of skim milk, 5 to 6 pieces of hard candy, or 1 tablespoon of sugar or honey. Wait 15 minutes and then re-check your blood glucose level. If it's still too low, take another 15 grams. Repeat these steps until your blood sugar is at least 70.

If you feel symptoms but can't check your blood glucose, treat yourself anyway rather than risk your glucose level going so low that you lose consciousness. If you do, someone will need to give you an injection of the hormone glucagon immediately. If you have a history of severe hypoglycemic episodes, your diabetes dream team will give you a prescription for an emergency dose and can teach family members and close friends how to inject it.

Hyperglycemia

High blood glucose or hyperglycemia, generally the result of insulin deficiency or insulin resistance, is what leads to all the long-term complications. But if your hyperglycemia is extremely high and goes untreated, it can be dangerous in the short term as well.

Several things cause hyperglycemia: if you have type 1 diabetes and you forget your insulin or don't give yourself enough insulin, or if the medications you take for type 2 diabetes don't lower your blood glucose enough. It might be because you ate more than you intended to eat or you were less active than you intended to be that day. Stresses on the body can cause your blood glucose to rise unexpectedly. The physical stress of a cold or flu, the emotional stress of a divorce, or the mental stress of work can all lead to higher than normal blood glucose. High levels of glucose in the blood will cause excessive thirst, increased urination, and an increased appetite. You'll also have glucose in your urine.

Checking your blood glucose often and adjusting diet and exercise will help keep your blood glucose normal. If your blood glucose tests high, you could exercise to lower it. (If it's above 250 and your urine has ketones, exercising could actually increase your blood glucose. Don't do it.) Cutting down on the amount of food you eat will also lower blood glucose. If these methods don't work, you need to discuss the possibility of adjusting your medication or insulin with your diabetes dream team. If you do not treat hyperglycemia when you first detect it, you could end up with a serious acute complication called ketoacidosis.

Ketoacidosis

Diabetic ketoacidosis or DKA is a condition that occurs when the body, not having enough insulin to use glucose for energy, starts burning fats. But fat isn't clean fuel; it leaves an acidic waste in your blood stream called ketones. Your body can get rid of some, but not all, of the ketones by excreting them in the urine. Eventually they'll build up—an acidic poison in the blood stream.

Most common in people with type 1 diabetes, this condition usually develops slowly, with symptoms similar to hyperglycemia. You'll notice you'll feel thirsty and your mouth is dry, and you're urinating more than usual. Your blood glucose levels and ketones in the urine will be high. As the condition worsens, symptoms include fatigue, dry and flushed skin, nausea, vomiting, abdominal pain, difficulty breathing, a fruity odor on the breath, and confusion. DKA can cause you to lose consciousness, and lead to coma and even death, so it must treated as a medical emergency. Call your doctor if your urine contains high ketones, especially high ketones in combination with high blood glucose or vomiting.

Hyperosmolar Hyperglycemic Nonketotic Syndrome (HHNS)

DKA is rare in individuals with type 2 diabetes, but they can develop another, similarly life-threatening condition known as hyperosmolar hyperglycemic nonketotic syndrome (HHNS). The kidney tries to help the body get rid of the excess blood glucose by flushing it out with so much urine you will eventually start to dehydrate. Urine production will slow down and urine will look very dark. You may also feel very thirsty. If you don't drink enough fluid, dehydration may become severe enough to cause seizures, coma, and eventually death.

Signs and symptoms of HHNS include a blood-sugar level greater than 600, a dry mouth, warm skin that does not sweat, fever over 101°F, sleepiness, confusion, loss of vision, hallucinations, and weakness on one side of the body. You will be extremely thirsty, but oddly enough, less so as the condition worsens. If you develop any of these symptoms, contact your doctor immediately; you'll need to go to the hospital for treatment right away.

Sick-Day Management

When you're ill—with a cold or flu or any kind of infection—your blood glucose can increase. Illness is stressful to the body, and the stress hormones that are released when you're sick cause the liver to produce more glucose, resulting in hyperglycemia. Minor illnesses can turn into the more serious conditions mentioned above, specifically DKA and HHNS. When you get sick, it's more important to keep your blood glucose in control—but it's also harder to do. That's why it's important to have a plan for those sick days. A plan prepared in advance can make getting a cold just a minor illness and not a life-threatening condition.

Making a sick day plan involves figuring out how often and when you should check your blood glucose and urine ketones, when you should call your diabetes dream team, foods to eat during this time, and how to take your medicines. You will also include important phone numbers so you can reach your diabetes dream team members quickly if illness strikes.

Making Your Sick Day Plan

The very nature of a plan is that you do it before you need it. So you want to work with your doctor and other members of your dream team ahead of time, so they can individualize the plan for you. Make an appointment to see your healthcare providers before you get sick. Here is a general guide to make your sick day plan:

▶ **Monitor more often**: Regardless of the type of diabetes you have, you will need to check your blood glucose and urine ketones more frequently than you normally check. If you have type 1 diabetes consider monitoring your blood glucose and urine ketones every four hours. In order to prevent DKA, you must check for ketones, too. If you have type 1, check every 4 hours. If you have type 2 diabetes, it's probably enough to monitor your blood glucose levels four times a day and only measure your urine ketone levels if your blood glucose levels go above 240.

▶ **Keep taking your diabetes medication.** You may not feel like eating much—you may not even be able to keep food on your stomach—but your blood glucose will rise just because you're sick. With type 1 diabetes, you might have to take more insulin than usual to bring your blood glucose levels down. If you are taking oral medication for type 2 diabetes, you may also need to use insulin for a brief time. In either case, your diabetes team will help you determine medication needs for your individualized sick day plan.

▶ **Drink plenty of fluids.** Water, warm unsweetened tea, and other unsweetened drinks help you get rid of the extra glucose in your blood while keeping you hydrated. You need to drink 8 ounces of water or calorie free fluid every hour you are awake.

▶ **Keep to your meal plan.** If consuming your usual fare is too difficult while you are ill, you can modify your meal plan. To keep your blood sugar steady, you should aim to get about 50 grams of carbohydrates every 3 to 4 hours. Consider saltine crackers, vanilla wafers, Lifesavers, graham crackers, dry toast, frozen yogurt, regular ice cream, Jello, sherbet, and applesauce—the regular versions, not sugar-free. If you can't hold down food, you have to drink clear liquids that contain sugar. Since you might get ill at any time, have some "regular" foods and beverages in your pantry, just in case.

▶ **Mind your medications.** When you are ill you might turn to an over-the-counter (OTC) medication to relieve your symptoms. However, many OTC medications contain sugar, alcohol, or other ingredients that will affect your blood glucose. Large doses of aspirin or any antibiotic may lower your blood glucose; decongestants and some cold and cough medications may raise it. Make sure you read all the warnings on the label as well as the list of ingredients. Ask your pharmacist to help you find medications that are sugar-free and safe to use. If you suffer from diabetes complications such as kidney disease or heart disease, ask your doctor before taking any over-the-counter medication.

▶ **Don't hesitate to call.** Dial your dream team when...

  ‣ You've been sick or had a fever for a couple of days without getting better.

  ‣ You've been vomiting or had diarrhea for longer than six hours.

  ‣ You have blood glucose higher than 240 after taking your extra insulin.

  ‣ You have blood glucose higher than 240 for more than 24 hours, though you've taken your oral diabetes medications.

⊳ You have moderate to large amounts of ketones in your urine.

⊳ You have any symptoms of DKA or dehydration such as feeling sleepier than usual, having trouble breathing, fuzzy thinking, fruity odor on your breath, or dry tongue and lips.

Long-Term Complications

Heart Disease and Stroke

Heart disease is the leading cause of diabetes-related deaths. Adults with diabetes have heart-disease-related death rates about two to four times higher than adults without diabetes. The risk for stroke is also 2 to 4 times higher among people with diabetes. A history of heart disease in your family increases your risk, leading to death in two out of every six people with diabetes. While you can't change the fact that diabetes or heart disease runs in your family, there are ways to ward off the damage.

▶ Lose the belly. If you're overweight and most of your weight is located in the abdominal area, you are at a greater risk for heart disease. Belly fat is associated with an increase production of LDL (bad) cholesterol. If your waist measures more than 40 inches for men and 35 inches for women, start a weight-loss and exercise plan.

▶ Control Cholesterol.

⊳ Lower LDL cholesterol. It causes narrowing and hardening of the arteries, so this number should be under 70 mg/dl.

⊳ Raise HDL cholesterol. It provides protection by removing deposits from inside the arteries. HDL for men should be above 40 mg/dl and for women above 50 mg/dl.

⊳ Lower Triglycerides. This "storage" form of fat can be elevated when diabetes is out of control. Triglycerides should be under 150 mg/dl.

▶ Decrease blood pressure. Hypertension makes your heart work harder to pump blood, straining the heart, damaging blood vessels, and increasing your risk of heart attack, stroke, eye disease, and kidney disease. Your blood pressure should be below 130/80.

▶ Kick the habit. Your risk for getting heart disease doubles if you are a smoker. Smoking narrows the blood vessels and increases the risk of other long term complication, such as eye disease and amputation.

Nephropathy—Diabetes Kidney Disease

Each year brings more than 4,000 new cases of end stage renal disease (ESRD)—kidney failure. Unfortunately, African-Americans are well represented in that number: Black folks with diabetes experience kidney failure about four times more often than white Americans with diabetes.

The kidneys use a system of delicate blood vessels to filter urine—getting rid of waste material while keeping nutrients and other cells that you need. When, as a result of diabetes, the kidneys are working harder to eliminate ketones and excess glucose, those tiny vessels can be damaged. Often there are no symptoms of kidney damage until you have lost 50 percent of your kidney function. This means your kidneys may be getting weaker and weaker without you realizing it. Eventually your very tired kidneys cannot keep up with the needs of the body. Once at this stage, you will require dialysis or a kidney transplant to stay alive. If you keep your blood sugar and blood pressure as close to normal as possible, you are less likely to develop this complication. Your doctor can detect early stages of kidney disease with routine blood and urine tests. Everyone with diabetes should have these tests at least once a year.

Retinopathy—Diabetes Eye Disease

Diabetes retinopathy is the most common diabetes eye disease. African-Americans are twice as likely to suffer from it as non-Hispanic whites. Retinopathy is caused by changes in the blood vessels of the retina, the lining in the back of the eye that senses light. You can imagine how delicate the blood vessels in the eye must be—and how easily damaged or clogged. If they are damaged, the body compensates by making new blood vessels. But the new ones are weak and prone to break and leak blood into the liquid in your eye causing you to see spots or "floaters." As the vessels break, scar tissue builds up, pulling the retina away from the wall of the eye. This is what causes blindness.

Laser therapy or vitrectomy can be used to prevent vision loss. Laser therapy helps to shrink the abnormal blood vessels in the eye. Vitrectomy is a surgical procedure that removes the blood that has leaked into your eye.

Diabetes is the leading cause of blindness in adults between the ages of 20 and 74. People with diabetes are also more likely to develop cataracts, a cloudiness that develops over the lens of the eye causing your vision to become impaired. They're also twice as likely to have glaucoma, a pressure that builds in the eye and presses on the optic nerve, causing peripheral blindness.

Everyone with diabetes should have a comprehensive dilated eye exam at least once a year. A dilated eye exam allows the doctor to widen your pupils and clearly see the inside of your eye.

You can prevent diabetes retinopathy by controlling blood sugar, blood pressure, and blood cholesterol. If you already have diabetes retinopathy, controlling blood sugar, blood pressure and blood cholesterol will slow down the progression of the disease. If you already have diabetes retinopathy, you may need to have an eye exam more often.

Nerve Damage Neuropathy

Nerves are the messengers in our body; they communicate pain, temperature, and other information between our body and the brain. They're nourished tiny blood vessels that are easily damaged by the effects of diabetes. There are two common types of nerve damage seen in diabetes.

Peripheral neuropathy or sensorimotor neuropathy causes tingling, pain, numbness, or weakness that often begins in the tips of the toes or fingers and gradually moves up to the feet and hands. Nerve damage in the feet makes them insensitive to pain, so you may have blisters, corns, or sores you don't even feel. Because diabetes slows healing, these minor injuries can become bigger infections that can spread to the bone and require amputation. African-Americans are much more likely to suffer lower limb amputation than white or Hispanic Americans with diabetes.

▷ Simple foot care and foot inspection can often prevent a minor cut from becoming the loss of limb.

▷ Check your feet every day for cuts, blisters, red spots, or swelling. See your doctor or podiatrist if you find any sores, blisters, or bruises.

▷ Wash feet every day with warm (not hot) water. Dry your feet thoroughly, especially between your toes.

▷ Apply lotion to keep your feet from cracking. Don't put it between the toes.

▷ Trim toe nails weekly. If you have trouble, have your doctor or podiatrist do it. They can smooth down corns and calluses, too.

▷ Do not walk barefoot. Wear shoes and socks whenever you are out; wear slippers at home.

▷ Protect your feet from hot and cold. Wear shoes at the beach and wear warm socks when out in the snow or cold.

▷ Keep blood flow to the feet by not crossing your legs for long periods of time. Put your feet up when sitting. Don't smoke. Also, be active.

The second common neuropathy is called *autonomic neuropathy*. This type of nerve damage causes problems with nerves that control the heart, blood pressure, digestion, respiration, and other internal organs. This type of nerve damage causes problems including:

▷ Damage to the nerves of the digestive tract—a disorder called gastroparesis that causes the stomach to hold its contents too long. It can causes heartburn, nausea, vomiting, feeling of fullness, weight loss, bloating, loss of appetite, and abdominal pain. Other complications of gastroparesis include bacterial overgrowth and the development of hardened masses of food that block the intestinal tract.

▷ Damage to the nerves that supply the bladder that can keep you from emptying your bladder completely, leading to bacterial infection and incontinence.

▷ Damage to nerves in the sexual organs, causing difficulty for both men and women to experience normal sexual response. In men, the nerve damage can cause erectile dysfunction. In women, it leads to difficulty with arousal, lubrication, and orgasm.

▷ Damage to the nerves that control sweating can make it difficult for the body to regulate temperature properly.

▷ Damage to the nerves of the pupils of the eye. The eye isn't as responsive to changes in light which may make a person have a difficult time driving in the dark.

▷ Damage to the nerves that control the heart and circulatory system, so the body can't adjust heart rate and blood pressure. For example, the heart won't slow down after you exercise, or your blood pressure might drop after sitting or standing, causing light-headedness and fainting.

People with diabetes are also more likely to suffer from other types of neuropathy including *proximal neuropathy*, pain in the thighs, hips, buttocks, or legs; and *focal neuropathy* that affects specific nerves in the head, torso, or leg. It can cause inability to focus the eye, double vision, aching behind the eye, Bell's palsy (paralysis on one side of the face), or pain in the front of the thigh, chest, stomach, shin, foot, or chest. The focal neuropathy is usually painful but will resolve over a few weeks or months.

Skin Problems

People with diabetes are more prone to bacterial infections of the eyelids (sties), hair follicles (boils), and deep skin tissues (carbuncles). When blood glucose levels are high, your body looses fluid which causes skin to become dry and crack; germs can enter through the cracks causing infection. People with diabetes are also more likely to suffer from fungal infections under the finger or toenails, jock itch, athlete's foot, and ringworm. Another problem is damage to the nerves in the sweat glands which can decrease the amount you sweat, making the skin dry and itchy. Drinking plenty of fluids is one of the many things you can do to help keep your skin moist and healthy.

Wash with mild soap, and dry completely. Check your skin after you wash. You want to be sure you have no dry, red, or sore spots that might get infected. Have your doctor recommend a good lotion. Wear all-cotton underwear. Tell your doctor or any member of your diabetes dream team about any skin problems you notice.

Gum and Tooth Problems

People with diabetes are more likely to suffer from gum disease because high glucose levels allow germs to grow more easily. The redness, soreness, and bleeding that result lead to a condition called periodontitis, an infection of the bone that supports the teeth. If you're over 45 and smoke, you're even more susceptible. Any gum or tooth infection will also raise your blood-sugar levels. Brushing, flossing, and visiting your dentist regularly will help prevent or control this condition. Also practice the following self-care actions:

> ⊳ Keep blood glucose as close to normal as possible.

> ⊳ Use dental floss at least once each day.

> ⊳ Brush your teeth after every meal and every snack.

> ⊳ If you wear false teeth, keep them clean.

▷ Call your dentist right away if you have problem with your teeth and gums.

▷ See your dentist at least twice a year and be sure to tell her you have diabetes.

▷ Stop smoking. Talk to your diabetes dream team about how to get help.

When you look at the possible complications of diabetes, you can see why having diabetes requires daily diligence. It is only your careful attention to your disease—taking the very best care of yourself—that will help keep these conditions at bay. The good news is that we know more than ever about how to treat and control the disease. That means that, if you make your plans and stick to your program, you focus on being healthy instead of fearing the worst.

Power Points

☞ Keeping blood glucose levels close to normal and controlling blood pressure and cholesterol can prevent or delay long-term diabetes complications.

☞ Complications include short term (acute) conditions and long-term (chronic) ones.

☞ Hypoglycemia is when your blood glucose level is below 70 and you are having symptoms including headaches, dizziness, and confusion. Treat it immediately with a fast acting source of carbohydrate (for example, 2 to 3 glucose tablets, 4 ounces of fruit juice, 4 ounces of regular soda, 1 cup of skim milk, 5 to 6 pieces of hard candy, or 1 tablespoon of sugar or honey).

☞ Symptoms of hyperglycemia—high blood glucose—are excessive thirst, increased urination, and increased appetite. Decreasing insulin levels through exercise or eating less can help.

☞ Chronic, long terms effects of diabetes include heart disease, stroke, kidney disease, and nerve damage.

☞ Having a cold, flu, or other infection can make diabetes symptoms worse. Work with your dream team to develop a written sick-day plan to help you cope with your illness without neglecting your diabetes.

Sick-Day Management Worksheets

IMPORTANT PHONE NUMBERS:

Doctor/clinic:_____

Daytime number:_____ After office/ clinic hours:_____

Diabetes educator:_____

Daytime number:_____ Diabetes educator after hours:_____

Emergency room:_____ Pharmacy:_____

Family or friend:_____ Number:_____

Making Contact:

I will contact someone on my dream team if:

▸ My blood sugar is higher than_____ for more than _____ hours.

▸ My urine ketone levels are_____ for more than _____ hours.

▸ I have had vomiting / diarrhea for longer than_____hours.

▸ I have trouble breathing, a fruity odor on my breath, or signs of dehydration.

▸ I am not sure what to do.

Other: _____

_____

MONITORING:

I will check my blood sugars every_____hours.

I will check my urine ketones when my blood sugar is higher than _____.

MEDICATIONS:

I will continue to take my oral medications and/or insulin unless: _____

_____

_____

I will adjust my insulin dosage by:_____

_____

OVER-THE-COUNTER MEDICATIONS:

Medications I can take include:_____

_____

_____

FOOD AND DRINK:

‣ If able to hold down fluids, I should drink 6 to 8 ounces of calorie-free beverages every hour.

‣ If I cannot handle my regular meal plan, I should consume 50 g carbohydrates from my modified food list every 3 to 4 hours (about 15 g carbohydrates an hour).

‣ If I am not able to keep down any food, I should drink 50 g carbohydrates from my clear liquid list every 3 to 4 hours (about 15 g carbohydrates an hour).

Modified food list:	Clear liquids with carbohydrates:
15 g carbohydrates	15 g carbohydrates
1/2 cup apple sauce	1 Popsicle (1 stick)
1/2 cup cooked cereal	4 oz. lemonade
4 oz. eggnog	3 tsp. honey add to decaf tea
8 oz. milk	5 Lifesavers candies
5 vanilla wafers	3 oz. grape juice
1 slice toast	4 oz. apple juice
1/2 cup regular ice cream	4 oz. regular soft drink (not diet, caffeine-free)
1/4 cup sherbet	1 cup sports drink
1 cup pastina	1/2 cup regular (not diet) gelatin
1/2 cup baked custard	1 cup broth soup
1/2 cup creamed soup	1/2 cup regular gelatin/Jell-O
1/3 cup fruit yogurt	
6 saltine crackers	
3 graham crackers	
1/2 cup frozen yogurt	
1/2 cup mashed potatoes	
1/4 cup regular pudding	

Time	Blood glucose/ Ketones	Temperature	Medicine Name and Dose	Food and Drink	Vomiting, Diarrhea, Urination	Other symptoms

Notes: _____

_____

_____

_____

_____

_____

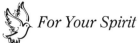 *For Your Spirit*

Bad Things, Good People

Why do bad things happen to good people? It's a question we often ask—especially during a tragedy such as the September 11 terrorist attacks or Hurricane Katrina, but also during a personal crisis such as the untimely death of a loved one or the diagnosis of a chronic disease. But the question assumes that bad things should only happen to bad people and that we live in a world where the righteous are exempt from facing troubles. Obviously neither is true.

The story of Job attempts to reach a real answer. You know Job. He did everything right—lived clean, prayed daily, followed the rules. He was a good husband, law-abiding citizen, and a spiritual leader. In his day, people believed in retribution—that good things happen to good people, and that if a bad thing occurred, it is because you did something wrong. So Job would have vigorously avoided doing bad things.

Certainly there are consequences for neglecting to do what's right. Those who suffer with diseases but refuse to properly care for their illness should expect things to grow progressively worse. But is the disease itself a punishment for some other misdeed? Difficulties in our lives aren't always due to bad behavior; sometimes things just happen and we must cope with them.

Job is our proof. In a flash and for no reason he knew about, he lost his livelihood, his home, and all ten of his children. But none of this swayed him until his own health began to fail. He wondered, just as we do, how a good God would allow the innocent to endure suffering. Dealing with his pain, loss, and public humiliation brought Job to an all time low, wishing that he had never been born: "And Job said, 'Let the day perish on which I was to be born, and the night which said, A boy is conceived'" (3:2-3).

A health crisis will do that to you—make you question God's reasons if not your own purpose on the planet. And it's especially hard when you have a chronic disease—something that can't be cured or is likely to grow progressively worse. Frankly, it's tiring to keep the faith in the face of trouble you know isn't going away.

But that is the point: keeping the faith. Job's true righteousness didn't come before he faced his tribulations, but after. The righteous are those who don't allow bad circumstances to alter their good character. You can truly claim your goodness only when you have persevered through trials and maintained your faith. Endurance is its own reward.

15 IN CLOSING: LIVING WITH DIABETES

Living with any chronic illness is "more than a notion," as the old folks used to say.

It's not just a matter of dealing with whatever physical problem you have. Chronic disease also requires discipline—to make the appointment, take the medicines, follow the doctors' advice, monitor your condition. You have to deal with the emotions that come with knowing that your body seems to have betrayed you. You have to cope with the fact that your life has changed permanently. This can leave you feeling overwhelmed and powerless, but you have to be able to find the faith to deal with a condition you didn't ask for and don't deserve—knowing that, somehow, everything is in Divine Order.

This is particularly true when it comes to living with diabetes, which can be so challenging physically, emotionally, and spiritually. Diabetes is not just a chronic disease, it's a daily disease. When you get up in the morning you have diabetes; when you go to bed at night you still have diabetes. You must make choices that will affect your diabetes and your life: monitor your glucose, take your pills, inject your insulin, read food labels, find time to exercise, put down the donut, check your weight, check your feet, hide the salt shaker. And you have to make those choices again tomorrow and the next day and the next.

But that's the good news: you can take it one day at a time. And over time you will learn how to nurture your body, your mind and your spirit so that you can have power over diabetes. You can live well with diabetes for life.

Nourishing the Body

Your physical being is at the foundation of your overall health. If you are ill, it is difficult to be mentally well and spiritually light. Research shows that dealing with chronic illness can literally make you depressed, and coping with your condition can cause you to lose faith and hope. So staying physically well is vital. Wellness requires the fitness triad—nutrition, exercise, and relaxation.

▶ Nutrition is the process of nourishing the body—and that means more than just putting something in your mouth. Food that nourishes is healthful, and it supports your diabetes meal plan is an important aspect of diabetes self management. Healthy eating will help you stay at a healthy weight, maintain good glucose control, lower blood pressure, and lower cholesterol levels. You should devote two to three hours daily towards preparing and eating your meals. Practice eating mindfully—paying attention to the flavors of your food instead of being consumed in TV, reading, or working. When you do other things while you eat, you are eating mindlessly, which can lead to overeating and making poor food choices.

▶ Physical activity is not only a good way to keep your bones and muscles strong, it burns extra calories to promote weight loss and lowers blood glucose levels. It's also a great way to relieve stress. Exercise releases endorphins that give you a feeling of well-being. Include aerobic exercise, strength training, and stretching into your weekly routine. And look for ways to get a little extra activity every day as part of your physical conditioning. Remember you don't need to do the 30 to 60 minutes of exercise all at once. Your exercise can be broken up into smaller segments throughout the day.

▶ Relaxation allows the physical body to regenerate itself. Aim for eight hours of sleep daily. Then, before you put anything else on your schedule, ink in one or two hours devoted to hobbies or leisure activity. A leisurely walk in the park or on the beach can be very relaxing. Others like to knit or listen to soft music. Many people just like to sit quietly and free their mind of all thoughts. It is important that you decide what helps you to relax and practice it daily. Relaxation can also help to keep your blood glucose levels in good control.

Feeding the Mind

The brain is that wrinkled-looking organ that is nestled in your skull. The mind is the seat of your ideas, thoughts, memories, feelings, and desires. The mind is synonymous with mental and emotional being. A healthy mind enables you to make sensible, sound judgments, based in objective reality. You can think prudently and make choices that will enable you to live well with diabetes. For example, if your mind is strong and you're thinking clearly, you are less likely to be subject to deniabetes. Thus you will make wiser choices about your self-care. However, if you haven't taken time to lay a strong foundation with the fitness triad (nutrition, exercise, and relaxation) your mental and emotional health will suffer. A healthy mind is dependent on a healthy body.

Elevating Your Spirit

The spirit is the home of the ideal self. It's at the spirit level that you experience your divine nature and manifest your highest moral strength. Prayer, meditation, and true worship foster a healthy spirit—and it's the fruit of that very prayer and meditation that aids in the healing of the mind and the body. African-Americans cling close to their spirituality—often taking part in daily prayer and renewal. Spirituality doesn't have to be connected to a particular religion or belief system; it can be the heart-connection you have with yourself, your beloved, and the world around you. But it does benefit you to have some kind of spiritual life. Research has shown that prayer and spirituality are associated with better health and longer life. However, if the body is broken or unbalanced, it will affect the mind and ultimately affect the spirit. So you see that the body, mind, and spirit operate as a continuum—literally a circle of life.

The Mind-Body Connection

You go out to dinner with friends. The restaurant you choose is known for its fried crab cakes appetizer, so everyone orders it. Fried chicken, candied yams, macaroni and cheese, collard greens with ham hocks, and good old-fashioned cornbread make up most of the entrees. You can't resist the temptation. You order a plate of wings with mac-and-cheese and string-beans seasoned with bacon. The cornbread that comes with it is the size of two decks of cards. On the way home that night you begin to feel very, very tired, your vision is blurred, and you have a terrible headache. When you walk into your front door, the children greet you with the usual noise and stories of the day's activities. It usually delights you, but today it just makes your head throb more. You ask them to be quiet, but of course they can't hush for long. Before you know it, you're yelling. When you realize what's happening the damage has already been done. You think to yourself, "I can't believe I yelled like that. Why did I overreact that way?"

Why *did* you act that way? You may be surprised to know that you hollered at your children because you went to dinner with your friends. Let's look at this scenario from the body, mind, and spirit prospective:

First, your food choices boosted your blood glucose, which led to the physical symptoms of fatigue, blurred vision, and headache. Your high blood glucose, in turn, affected you mentally. You couldn't feel the pleasure your children normally bring you. You lost control of your emotions and snapped at them instead. Your head was only filled with the ache, not prayerful thoughts. Spiritually, you lost the connection between you and your children—at least momentarily—and you feel like a dishonorable parent.

So there you see the connections between the mind, body, and soul—and how subtly they can affect one another.

Wellness is more than being free from disease. It is when your entire being—the vessel and the spirit—is functioning on the highest levels. But to keep that balance is a challenge—especially when you are dealing with diabetes. Your goal is to make progress "One Day at a Time."

No one is perfect and diabetes by it's very nature is unpredictable. There will be days when you eat something that you know you probably shouldn't, and have to face the consequences. And there will be days when you've done everything "right" and, still, your blood glucose levels will be higher than expected. Don't be discouraged. Make a note in your log book to discuss it with your diabetes dream team at your next visit. Then move on. "Yesterday is gone" and you can't rewind time.

It is only then that one can experience true spirituality. Conversely, when one is experiencing true spirituality, the mind is clear and they are led to make better health choices resulting in positive outcomes.

Only Human

The song "One Day at a Time" reminds us that we're only human, and as a human, you will experience many emotions as you live with diabetes. It's natural to move back and forth between acceptance, fear, resentment, frustration, and depression. Allow yourself to feel and express your feelings. And in between, find a way to take care of yourself—your whole self.

Ask for help if you find you can't seem to get back on track. Talk to family, friends, the clergy, or any member of your diabetes dream team to motivate you back to positive action.

Learn to cope with stress. Everyone has it in their lives. When you have diabetes, stress can affect your ability to control the disease. Embracing your spirituality can reduce stress, because it allows you to turn diabetes over to your higher power and know that you are not carrying the burden alone.

Recognize the demands of diabetes. Accept the work of monitoring and treating your condition. Learn to adapt and make healthy food substitutions and modifications, so that you can continue to enjoy family meals and traditional holiday get-togethers.

Nurture yourself with things that are enjoyable for you. Diabetes may limit the number of sweets you can eat, but it doesn't have to take the sweetness out of your life. Treat yourself to a massage or pedicure, a concert ticket, a visit to a good friend.

Fill your mind with information. Educate yourself and keep abreast of new information regarding diabetes self management. The more you know, the more it will seem like second-nature to you.

Don't make diabetes your enemy. Think of it as your companion that will travel with you on the journey to the rest of your life. You are not a diabetic. You are a person full of life, with hopes and dreams—and you happen to have diabetes.

Appendix A

Sample Menus

In this section, you will find a two-week sample menu chock full of Caribbean and traditional southern meal time favorites. Many newly diagnosed people find it easier to follow sample menus than to have to figure out what to eat at each meal. Once you get used to your new meal plan, it will become second nature and these sample menus will be a memory.

Everything on the menu won't appeal to you. If you don't like a particular food on the menu, simply substitute a food of similar value. You will notice that the carbohydrate values for each food item have been noted to make it easy for carbohydrate counting.

Day 1

Breakfast

1 cup grits	30
1 large egg, scrambled	0
1 slice 100% whole wheat bread, toasted	15
1/2 cup orange juice	15
1 teaspoon margarine	0
Beverage, coffee, brewed	0
Sugar substitute—Splenda	0
1 fl. oz. milk, skim or nonfat	0
Total	60

Lunch

1 slice pizza (1/8 of 12″ pie)	30
Mixed salad	
1 cup lettuce, romaine, raw	5
1/2 cup tomato, red, ripe, sliced	3
1 Tbsp. Italian salad dressing, regular	0
1 cup diced cantaloupe, raw	15
No calorie beverage	0
Total	53

Dinner

4 oz. **Escoveitch Fish**	8
1 **West Indian Plantain Cake**	29
1 cup **Sautéed Callaloo**	10
1/2 mango, raw	15
No calorie beverage	0
Total	62

Snack 1

6 saltine crackers, fat free	15
1 tsp. peanut butter, smooth	0
No calorie beverage	0
Total	15

Day 2

Breakfast

3/4 cup Cheerios cereal	15
1 cup fortified soy milk	15
1 medium (7" long) banana, raw	30
Beverage, coffee, brewed	0
1 fl. oz. fortified soy milk	0
Sugar substitute	0
Total	60

Lunch

2 slices 7-grain bread	30
Tuna salad	
3 oz. light tuna fish, canned in water	0
1 Tbsp. mayonnaise, reduced calorie or diet	0
2 iceberg lettuce leaves, raw	0
2 thin slices red onions, raw	0
1 1/4 cup watermelon	15
No calorie beverage	0
Total	45

Dinner

Caribbean Chili and Sweet potatoes	
1/2 cup bean mixture + 1/4 potato	26
Good-for-You Cornbread (1 square)	23
1/2 cup juice packed pineapple	15
No calorie beverage	0
Total	64

Snack 1

3/4 cup cherry yogurt, nonfat, sweetened with low-calorie sweetener	15
No calorie beverage	0
Total	15

Day 3

Breakfast

2 turkey sausage patties (2 oz each)	0
2 **Buttermilk Biscuits**	26
Tropical fruit salad	
1 cup papaya, peeled, cubed	15
1 guava, raw	8
Beverage, coffee, brewed	0
1 fl .oz. milk, skim or nonfat	0
Sugar substitute	0
Total	49

Lunch

1 cup **Black-Eyed Pea and Mushroom Soup**	20
1 French roll	20
1 cup mixed salad	
1 cup lettuce, romaine, 1/2 cup tomato	8
1 Tbsp. vinaigrette salad dressing	0
1 fresh apple	15
No calorie beverage	0
Total	63

Dinner

4 oz. ham, fresh, cooked, lean only	0
1 small sweet potato, baked in skin, no salt	12
1/2 cup turnip greens	5
1 small roll	15
1 tsp. margarine	0
1/2 cup applesauce, unsweetened	15
No calorie beverage	0
Total	47

Snack 1

6 Triscuit crackers, 100% whole wheat	15
2 thin slices turkey, light meat	0
Total	15

Day 4

Breakfast

1 cup oatmeal	25
1/2 cup milk, skim or nonfat	6
1 small (2") peach, raw	8
1 slice 100% whole wheat bread, toasted	15
1 tsp. margarine	0
Beverage, coffee, brewed	0
1 fl oz. milk, skim or nonfat	0
sugar substitute	0
Total	54

Lunch

4 oz. **Turkey Burger**	0
Cucumber salad	
1/2 cup sliced cucumber, raw	5
1 Tbsp. vinigarette dressing	0
1 whole wheat hamburger bun	22
1 cup **Summer Breeze Smoothie**	33
No calorie beverage	0
Total	60

Dinner

4 oz. **Cornmeal Crusted Catfish**	20
Orzo and snap peas	
3/4 cup cooked orzo	30
1 tsp. olive oil	0
1/2 cup sugar snap peas	5
No calorie beverage	0
Total	55

Snack 1

Trail mix	
3/4 oz. pretzels, hard, bite size	15
10 peanuts, dry roasted, salted	0
No calorie beverage	0
Total	15

Day 5

Breakfast

1/4 cup Egg Beaters egg substitute	0
1 English muffin, 100% whole wheat, toasted	25
1 tsp. margarine	0
2 tsp. strawberry jelly sweetened with artificial sweetener	5
3/4 cup pineapple, canned in juice	21
Beverage, coffee, brewed	0
1 fl. oz. milk, skim or nonfat	0
Sugar substitute	0
Total	51

Lunch

1 1/2 cup **Lawrence's Cajun Style Gumbo**	12
1/2 cup long grain rice	23
1 oz. roll, 100% whole wheat	15
3 small apricots, raw	15
No calorie beverage	0
Total	65

Dinner

4 oz. beef steak, broiled	0
Sautéed mushrooms and onions	
1/4 cup mushrooms, sautéed	3
1/4 cup onions, yellow, sautéed	2
2 tsp. oil, vegetable, canola	0
1/2 small (1 3/4" to 2 1/2") white potato, baked	15
2 Tbsp. sour cream, reduced fat	0
1/2 cup asparagus, cooked	5
1 tsp. margarine	0
1 slice **Mock-Southern Sweet Potato Pie**	24
No calorie beverage	0
Total	49

Snack 1

3 (2 1/2") graham crackers	10
1/2 cup milk, skim or nonfat	6
Total	16

Day 6

Breakfast

1 small (2 oz) Lenders Bagel, toasted	30
2 Canadian bacon	0
3 egg whites, scrambled	0
1 fresh orange (medium)	15
Beverage, coffee, brewed	0
1 fl. oz. milk, skim or nonfat	0
Sugar substitute	0
Total	45

Lunch

Salmon salad	
3 oz. pink salmon, canned	0
2 egg whites, cooked	0
1/2 tsp. cayenne pepper	0
1/2 cup sliced cucumber	2
1 Tbsp. mayonnaise, reduced-calorie or diet	0
1 wedge lemon juice	0
1 medium (2 oz) cracked wheat roll	15
1 kiwi fruit mixed with	12
1 cup strawberries, slices	15
No calorie beverage	0
Total	44

Dinner

4 oz. **Mango Pork**	27
1/2 cup white rice, long grain	20
1 cup **Down Home Collard Greens**	10
1/2 cup Jello, unsweetened	0
No calorie beverage	0
Total	57

Snack 1

Nachos	
10 tortilla chips, light (baked with less oil)	12
1 oz. cheddar cheese, low fat	0
1/4 cup salsa	3
No calorie beverage	0
Total	15

Day 7

Breakfast

1 piece **Good-for-You Cornbread**	23
1 tsp. margarine	0
1 oz. cheddar cheese, low fat	0
1/2 cup peach, canned in juice	15
Beverage, coffee, brewed	0
1 fl. oz. milk, skim or nonfat	0
Sugar substitute	0
Total	38

Lunch

3 oz. **Home-style Meat Loaf**	3
1/2 cup mashed potato	15
1 tsp. margarine	0
1 fl. oz. milk, skim or nonfat	15
1/2 cup peas and carrots	5
1 medium pear, raw	15
No calorie beverage	0
Total	60

Dinner

1 1/2 cups **Old Fashion Beef Stew**	18
1/2 cup noodles	15
1/2 cup three bean salad (green, wax, and kidney)	5
1 slice (1/12 cake) **Upside Down Pineapple Cake** in a pan	21
No calorie beverage	0
Total	59

Snack 1

1/2 cup vanilla pudding, sugar free	5
No calorie beverage	0
Total	5

Day 8

Breakfast

2 (4-inch) homade buttermilk pancakes	15
2 Tbsp. lite pancake syrup	15
3/4 cup vanilla yogurt, low fat	15
1 1/4 cup strawberries	15
Beverage, coffee, brewed	0
1 fl. oz. milk, skim or nonfat	0
Sugar substitute	0
Total	60

Lunch

Shrimp salad	
3 oz. shrimp, steamed or boiled	0
1 egg white, cooked	0
1 small stalk celery	0
1 Tbsp. mayonnaise, reduced calorie	0
1 medium pumpernickel roll	20
1 large (4 1/2") carambola (starfruit)	10
1 cup lettuce	2
1 cup cherry tomato	7
1 Tbsp. thousand island dressing, reduced calorie	0
1 cup sliced sweet red pepper	5
No calorie beverage	0
Total	44

Dinner

3 oz. **Crispy Oven Fried Chicken** (1/2 breast or 2 small legs)	6
1 cup **Sweet Potato Casserole**	34
1/2 cup string beans	5
1 tsp. margarine	
1/2 cup chocolate frozen yogurt, sugar free, fat free	15
No calorie beverage	0
Total	60

Snack 1

1/2 small (6 inches) banana, mashed and mixed with	15
2 tsp. peanut butter, reduced-fat on	0
1/2 English muffin, 100% whole wheat	15
Total	30

Day 9

Breakfast

Western omelet	
3 egg whites	0
1/4 cup sweet green pepper, chopped	2
1/4 cup onions, chopped	5
1/2 cup grits	15
1 **Buttermilk Biscuit**	15
1 tsp. margarine	0
17 grapes	6
Beverage, coffee, brewed	0
1 fl. oz. milk, skim or nonfat	0
Total	43

Lunch

Grilled cheese with mango salsa	
2 slices 100% whole wheat bread	30
3 oz. Swiss cheese, low fat	0
Mango salsa	
1/2 cup mango, peeled, chopped	15
1 wedge fresh lime juice	0
1/4 cup red onions, chopped	3
1/4 cup sweet red pepper	2
Cooking spray	0
1 Tbsp. honey mustard dressing	5
6 fl. oz. Vegetable Juice, V-8	5
Total	60

Dinner

3 oz. **Cumin Roast Goat**	5
1/2 cup boiled potato	15
3/4 cup kale, cooked	5
1 tsp. olive oil	0
1/4 cup onions, chopped	3
1/2 cup homemade bread pudding	30
No calorie beverage	0
Total	58

Snack 1

1 oz. (22 nuts) almonds, dry roasted	0
2 cups microwave popcorn, low fat, low sodium	15
Total	15

Day 10

Breakfast

3/4 cup cereal, Kellogg's Raisin Bran	30
1 cup milk, skim or nonfat	12
Beverage, coffee, brewed	0
1 fl oz. milk, skim or nonfat	0
Sugar substitute	0
Total	42

Lunch

1 multigrain roll	20
3 oz. pork, shredded, lean, roasted	0
1 Tbsp. barbeque sauce	5
1/3 cup baked beans	15
1 cup homemade coleslaw	15
No calorie beverage	0
Total	55

Dinner

1 cup **Haitian Legume**	22
2/3 cup rice	30
2 Tbsp. **Pickliz**	3
Tossed salad	
1 cup romaine lettuce, raw	5
1/4 cup tomato, red, ripe	3
1 Tbsp. French dressing, reduced calorie	
Total	53

Snack 1

1/2 cup cottage cheese, low fat	3
9 baby carrots, raw	7
No calorie beverage	0
Total	10

Day 11

Breakfast

2 Salmon cakes	7
1/4 cup scrambled egg, made from Egg Beaters	0
1 cup grits	30
1 cup raspberries	15
Beverage, coffee, brewed	0
1 fl oz. milk, skim or nonfat	0
sugar substitute	0
Total	52

Lunch

1 cup **Easy Rice and Beans**	47
Tossed salad	
1 cup romaine lettuce, raw	5
1/2 cup tomato, red, ripe, sliced	3
1 Tbsp. salad dressing, Italian, regular	0
1/2 cup vanilla ice cream, light, w/aspartame, no sugar	15
No calorie beverage	0
Total	70

Dinner

3 oz. beef brisket, slices	0
1/2 cup white potato, boiled, with peel	15
1 tsp. margarine	0
1/2 cup spinach	5
3/4 cup **Southern Banana Pudding**	33
No calorie beverage	0
Total	53

Snack 1

1 rice cake topped with	5
1/4 cup ricotta cheese, part skim	3
1/4 cup salsa	3
No calorie beverage	0
Total	11

Day 12

Breakfast

French toast	
2 slices whole wheat bread	30
1/4 cup egg substitute	0
1/2 cup skim milk	6
1 tsp. vanilla extract flavoring	0
1 medium (7 inches) banana, sliced	30
1/2 oz. (7 halves) walnuts, chopped	0
Beverage, coffee, brewed	0
1 fl. oz. milk, skim or nonfat	0
Sugar substitute	0
Total	**66**

Lunch

Chicken salad	
4 oz. chicken, breast, no skin, roasted	0
1 Tbsp. mayonnaise, reduced calorie	0
1 small (5 inches) celery	0
1 oz. slivered almonds, dry roasted, without salt	5
1 wedge fresh lemon juice	0
1 medium oatmeal roll	15
2 (2 1/2") nectarines	30
No calorie beverage	0
Total	50

Dinner

Shrimp Creole	
4 oz. shrimp, sauté	0
1 tsp. Creole Seasoning	0
1 tsp. oil, vegetable, canola	0
1 medium (5" long) corn on cob	20
1 tsp. margarine	0
1 cup (1-inch pieces) chayote/christophine fruit, boiled	8
1/2 cup homemade rice pudding	30
No calorie beverage	0
Total	58

Snack 1

17 seedless grapes	6
1 oz. cheese, cheddar or Colby, low fat	0
Total	6

Day 13

Breakfast

2 (4-inch) waffle, plain, low fat	30
1 Tbsp. pancake syrup, reduced calorie	5
1 tsp. margarine	0
6 oz. fruit yogurt, nonfat, sweetened w/low calorie sweetener	15
1/2 small (3 1/2-inch diameter) grapefruit	8
Sugar substitute	0
Beverage, coffee, brewed	0
1 fl. oz. milk, skim or nonfat	0
Sugar substitute	0
Total	58

Lunch

2 slices bread, rye	30
3 oz. roast beef, sliced	0
1 tsp. mayonnaise, reduced calorie	0
1/2 cup macaroni or pasta salad	15
1/2 cup fruit cocktail, canned in juice	15
No calorie beverage	0
Total	60

Dinner

4 oz. chicken, broiler or fryer, leg, no skin, roasted	0
1 small sweet potato, baked in skin	15
1 cup broccoli, cooked	5
1/8 of 9-inch pie cherry, with one crust	40
No calorie beverage	0
Total	60

Snack 1

1/2 cup Cheerios cereal	10
1/2 cup milk, skim or nonfat	6
No calorie beverage	0
Total	16

Day 14

Breakfast

Grilled peanut butter and banana	
2 slices 100% whole wheat bread	30
2 Tbsp. smooth peanut butter, reduced fat	0
1 small (6-inch) banana	15
Cooking spray	0
Beverage, coffee, brewed	0
1 fl. oz. milk, skim or nonfat	0
Sugar substitute	0
Total	45

Lunch

Smoked turkey wrap	
1 tortilla, whole wheat	15
1 Tbsp. cream cheese, low fat mixed with	0
1 clove garlic	0
4 oz. turkey breast, smoked, sliced	0
1 thin slice turkey bacon, cooked	0
2 arugula leaves	0
3 thin slices onions, red onions	2
1 large (3 1/4-inch) apple w/skin	30
No calorie beverage	0
Total	47

Dinner

3 oz. roast chicken	0
2/3 cup brown rice	30
1 cup **Spicy Okra**	10
1/2 cup **Southern Banana Pudding**	22
No calorie beverage	0
Total	62

Snack 1

3/4 cup blueberry yogurt, nonfat milk, sweetened	
with low-calorie sweetener	15
No calorie beverage	0
Total	15

APPENDIX B

RECIPES

The pages that follow include select recipes from the sample menus. Each recipe has been analyzed for nutrient totals and includes a nutrient facts label. The label will help you to better understand how a serving of that recipe fits into your daily meal plan. You can also use it to help adjust your portion sizes based on your carbohydrate goals, and to manage your other nutrition goals for fat, cholesterol and sodium intake. If you're not sure how to work a recipe into your personal meal plan, take it to your dietitian for help.

Each recipe has also been tested for deliciousness. But deliciousness is in the taste buds of the beholder. You may want to adjust ingredients to suit your taste. That may mean adding more garlic and less onion, or switching marjoram for the basil. Feel free to tweak the recipes with spices you like; they don't add calories or carbs. Just watch the salt—including seasoned salt and spice blends that contain salt. You don't want to add sodium to your food.

Side Dishes and Seasonings

Main Dishes

Sweets

Side Dishes and Seasonings

Buttermilk Biscuits

Olive oil for coating pan
1 cup all-purpose or Nutriblend flour
2 tsp. baking powder
1 tsp. sugar
1/8 tsp. baking soda
1/8 tsp. sea salt
1 Tbsp. butter
1/3 cup low-fat buttermilk
1/4 cup non-fat or low-fat plain yogurt
Flour for the surface to cut out biscuits

Pre-heat oven to 425°F. Wipe 8-inch round baking pan with oil and set aside.

In a medium size bowl mix the flour, baking powder, baking soda, sugar, and sea salt. Using a pastry blender or by hand, cut the butter into the flour mixture until it becomes crumbles. Stir yogurt and buttermilk into flour mixture with a fork until just moistened. Place dough onto a lightly floured cutting board. Sprinkle with a small amount of flour and shape dough into a disk. With a rolling pin, pat out the dough until it is about 1/2 inch thick. Cut out biscuits with a 2 1/2-inch round cookie cutter. Use prepared 8-inch round baking pan. Place biscuits in prepared cake pan.
Bake for 10 to 12 minutes until biscuits are cooked in the middle and golden brown on bottom.

Makes 8 servings

Recipe courtesy Chef Marc Anthony Bynum.

Nutrition Facts

Serving Size 1 biscuit (38g)
Servings Per Container 8

Amount Per Serving

Calories 90	Calories from Fat 30

% Daily Value*

Total Fat 3.5g	5%
Saturated Fat 1.5g	8%
Trans Fat 0g	
Cholesterol 5mg	2%
Sodium 210mg	9%
Total Carbohydrate 13g	4%
Dietary Fiber 0g	0%
Sugars 2g	
Protein 2g	

Vitamin A 2%	•	Vitamin C 0%
Calcium 6%	•	Iron 4%

*Percent Daily Values are based on a 2,000 calorie diet. Your daily values may be higher or lower depending on your calorie needs:

		Calories:	2,000	2,500
Total Fat	Less than		65g	80g
Saturated Fat	Less than		20g	25g
Cholesterol	Less than		300mg	300mg
Sodium	Less than		2,400mg	2,400mg
Total Carbohydrate			300g	375g
Dietary Fiber			25g	30g

Calories per gram:
Fat 9 • Carbohydrate 4 • Protein 4

Good-for-You Cornbread

1 cup cornmeal
1 cup flour
1/4 cup sugar
1 tsp. baking powder
1 cup low-fat (1%) buttermilk
1 egg, whole
1/4 cup margarine, regular, tub
1 teaspoon vegetable oil (to grease
    baking pan)

Preheat oven to 350°F.

Mix together cornmeal, flour, sugar, and baking powder.

In another bowl, combine buttermilk and egg. Beat lightly. Slowly add buttermilk and egg mixture to dry ingredients. Add margarine and mix by hand or with mixer for 1 minute.

Bake for 20 to 25 minutes in an 8" × 8", greased baking dish. Cool. Cut into 10 even squares.

Makes 10 servings

Recipe from National Institute of Health, Heart Healthy Home Cooking.

Nutrition Facts

Serving Size 1 square (65g)
Servings Per Container 10

Amount Per Serving

Calories 160   Calories from Fat 60

% Daily Value*

Total Fat 6g	**9%**
Saturated Fat 1.5g	**8%**
Trans Fat 0g	
Cholesterol 25mg	**8%**
Sodium 125mg	**5%**
Total Carbohydrate 23g	**8%**
Dietary Fiber 2g	**8%**
Sugars 5g	
Protein 4g	

Vitamin A 4%	•	Vitamin C 0%
Calcium 6%	•	Iron 6%

*Percent Daily Values are based on a 2,000 calorie diet. Your daily values may be higher or lower depending on your calorie needs:

		Calories:	2,000	2,500
Total Fat	Less than		65g	80g
Saturated Fat	Less than		20g	25g
Cholesterol	Less than		300mg	300mg
Sodium	Less than		2,400mg	2,400mg
Total Carbohydrate			300g	375g
Dietary Fiber			25g	30g

Calories per gram:
  Fat 9 • Carbohydrate 4 • Protein 4

Sweet Potato Casserole

3 oranges
1/2 cup brown sugar, Splenda blend
1/4 cup brandy
1/4 cup nonfat/skim evaporated milk
2 Tbsp. margarine
1/2 tsp. salt
Pinch of black pepper
3 medium sweet potatoes (boiled and
    mashed)
Pinch ground nutmeg

Preheat oven to 350°F.

Zest 1 orange and set aside.

Scoop pulp out of all oranges and drain in a large bowl. Add brown sugar, Splenda blend to the pulp.

In a pan heat brandy, evaporated milk, margarine, salt, and pepper. Add the sweet potatoes, orange pulp, orange zest, and nutmeg. Mix well.

Place mixture in a casserole dish and bake for about 20-30 minutes.

Makes 8 servings.

Recipe courtesy Marlisa Brown, RD, and Constance Brown-Riggs, RD, aka "Soul Sisters Cook." This recipe takes sweet potatoes to a whole "nutha" level.

Nutrition Facts

Serving Size 1/2 (110g)
Servings Per Container 8

Amount Per Serving

Calories 110   Calories from Fat 25

% Daily Value*

Total Fat 3g	**5%**
Saturated Fat 0.5g	**3%**
Trans Fat 0g	
Cholesterol 0mg	**0%**
Sodium 200mg	**8%**
Total Carbohydrate 17g	**6%**
Dietary Fiber 2g	**8%**
Sugars 8g	
Protein 2g	

Vitamin A 190% • Vitamin C 25%

Calcium 4% • Iron 2%

*Percent Daily Values are based on a 2,000 calorie diet. Your daily values may be higher or lower depending on your calorie needs:

		Calories:	2,000	2,500
Total Fat	Less than		65g	80g
Saturated Fat	Less than		20g	25g
Cholesterol	Less than		300mg	300mg
Sodium	Less than		2,400mg	2,400mg
Total Carbohydrate			300g	375g
Dietary Fiber			25g	30g

Calories per gram:
  Fat 9 • Carbohydrate 4 • Protein 4

Down Home Collard Greens

Cooking spray

1 (4-oz.) smoked turkey leg or turkey ham

2 lbs. collard greens washed and cut into 2" pieces

4 cups reduced-sodium chicken broth

2 Tbsp. minced garlic

2 tsp. onion powder

Pinch red pepper flakes

Black pepper to taste

Vinegar to taste

Spray large soup pot with cooking spray. Heat over medium heat until hot. Add turkey leg and cook for 2–3 minutes, turning occasionally.

Add collards, broth, garlic, onion powder, pepper flakes, black pepper, and vinegar.

Cover. Cook 2 1/2 hours, stirring occasionally.

Makes 10 servings

Recipe courtesy of Marlisa Brown, RD and Constance Brown-Riggs, RD, aka "Soul Sisters Cook."

Nutrition Facts

Serving Size 1 cup (201g)

Servings Per Container 10

Amount Per Serving

Calories 80	Calories from Fat 20

	% Daily Value*
Total Fat 2.5g	4%
Saturated Fat 0.5g	3%
Trans Fat 0g	
Cholesterol 20mg	7%
Sodium 180mg	8%
Total Carbohydrate 6g	2%
Dietary Fiber 3g	12%
Sugars 0g	
Protein 7g	

Vitamin A 120%	•	Vitamin C 50%
Calcium 15%	•	Iron 2%

*Percent Daily Values are based on a 2,000 calorie diet. Your daily values may be higher or lower depending on your calorie needs:

		Calories:	2,000	2,500
Total Fat	Less than		65g	80g
Saturated Fat	Less than		20g	25g
Cholesterol	Less than		300mg	300mg
Sodium	Less than		2,400mg	2,400mg
Total Carbohydrate			300g	375g
Dietary Fiber			25g	30g

Calories per gram:

Fat 9 • Carbohydrate 4 • Protein 4

Spicy Okra

2 10-oz. packages frozen, cut okra
1 tsp. vegetable oil
1 medium onion, coarsely chopped
1 14-1/2-oz. can of diced tomatoes
1 fresh jalapeno pepper
    (or habanero chile), pierced 3 time
    with fork
1/2 tsp. salt
1/4 tsp. black pepper

Rinse okra in a colander under hot
water.

Heat oil in a 10-inch heavy skillet over
moderately high heat. Sauté onion
for about 3 minutes. Add tomatoes
(including juice) and chili. Boil.

Stir the mixture for 8 minutes. Add okra
and cook, gently stirring, until okra is
tender (about 5 minutes).

Stir in salt and pepper and discard the
chili.

Makes 5 servings

Recipe from National Institute of Health,
Heart Healthy Home Cooking.

Nutrition Facts

Serving Size 1 cup (234g)
Servings Per Container 5

Amount Per Serving

Calories 100   Calories from Fat 25

                                        % Daily Value*

Total Fat 3g	**5%**
Saturated Fat 0.5g	**3%**
Trans Fat 0g	
Cholesterol 0mg	**0%**
Sodium 290mg	**12%**
Total Carbohydrate 15g	**5%**
Dietary Fiber 4g	**16%**
Sugars 7g	
Protein 2g	

Vitamin A 15%   •   Vitamin C 35%

Calcium 10%   •   Iron 4%

*Percent Daily Values are based on a 2,000 calorie
diet. Your daily values may be higher or lower
depending on your calorie needs:

		Calories:	2,000	2,500
Total Fat	Less than		65g	80g
Saturated Fat	Less than		20g	25g
Cholesterol	Less than		300mg	300mg
Sodium	Less than		2,400mg	2,400mg
Total Carbohydrate			300g	375g
Dietary Fiber			25g	30g

Calories per gram:
    Fat 9 • Carbohydrate 4 • Protein 4

Braised Cabbage

1/4 cup blended oil
1 small red onion sliced
1/4 cup brown sugar
1 lb. red cabbage
1 oz. red wine vinegar
1 cup red wine
1 cup orange juice
1 stick cinnamon

Heat oil in pan on stove top. Add red onion and sweat till translucent. Add brown sugar till caramelized. Then add apples and deglaze with vinegar.

Bring to a boil, and then add red wine, orange juice, and cinnamon stick. Let simmer for 5 minutes.

Add cabbage to mixture and let cook on the stove top for 10 minutes. Then cover with foil and place in 350°F oven for 20 minutes till tender. Remove, adjust seasoning, and serve.

Makes 8 servings.

Courtesy Chef Marc Anthony Bynum.

Nutrition Facts

Serving Size 1 cup (203g)
Servings Per Container 8

Amount Per Serving

Calories 140	Calories from Fat 60

	% Daily Value*
Total Fat 7g	11%
Saturated Fat 0.5g	3%
Trans Fat 0g	
Cholesterol 0mg	0%
Sodium 30mg	1%
Total Carbohydrate 15g	5%
Dietary Fiber 3g	12%
Sugars 9g	
Protein 2g	

Vitamin A 25%	•	Vitamin C 120%
Calcium 6%	•	Iron 6%

*Percent Daily Values are based on a 2,000 calorie diet. Your daily values may be higher or lower depending on your calorie needs:

		Calories:	2,000	2,500
Total Fat	Less than		65g	80g
Saturated Fat	Less than		20g	25g
Cholesterol	Less than		300mg	300mg
Sodium	Less than		2,400mg	2,400mg
Total Carbohydrate			300g	375g
Dietary Fiber			25g	30g

Calories per gram:
Fat 9 • Carbohydrate 4 • Protein 4

Sautéed Callaloo

2 lbs. callaloo leaves
1 Tbsp. margarine
1/4 tsp. salt
pinch of black pepper
1 medium diced onion
1 hot chili pepper, sliced
1 clove minced garlic

Thoroughly wash the fresh callaloo, discarding old leaves and the seeds at the top. Chop into small pieces and drain. Heat the margarine until melted. Add onions and well drained callaloo. Add chili pepper and garlic. Mix thoroughly. Cover and cook on a low flame until tender. Serve immediately.

Makes 5 servings

This recipe is from Leslene Gordon, PhD, RD. Callaloo is cooked by itself or with salted codfish. It is the main ingredient in the Jamaican pepper pot soup, not to be confused with the Easter Caribbean callaloo soup which is made with the leaves of the dasheen plant.

Nutrition Facts	
Serving Size 1 cup (216g)	
Servings Per Container 5	
Amount Per Serving	
Calories 80	Calories from Fat 25
	% Daily Value*
Total Fat 3g	**5%**
Saturated Fat 0.5g	**3%**
Trans Fat 0g	
Cholesterol 0mg	**0%**
Sodium 170mg	**7%**
Total Carbohydrate 10g	**3%**
Dietary Fiber 1g	**4%**
Sugars 1g	
Protein 5g	
Vitamin A 110% • Vitamin C 170%	
Calcium 40% • Iron 25%	

*Percent Daily Values are based on a 2,000 calorie diet. Your daily values may be higher or lower depending on your calorie needs:

		Calories:	2,000	2,500
Total Fat	Less than		65g	80g
Saturated Fat	Less than		20g	25g
Cholesterol	Less than		300mg	300mg
Sodium	Less than		2,400mg	2,400mg
Total Carbohydrate			300g	375g
Dietary Fiber			25g	30g

Calories per gram:
Fat 9 • Carbohydrate 4 • Protein 4

Black-Eyed Pea and Mushroom Soup

1 tablespoon olive oil
1 medium chopped onion, yellow
1 cup sliced mushrooms
2 medium celery stalks
2 medium carrots
1 Tbsp. minced garlic
1/2 tsp. dried thyme
1 15-oz. can black-eyed peas
2 10.5-oz. cans low-sodium chicken broth
1/2 tsp. black pepper

Heat olive oil in a large pot over medium heat.

Sauté onions until translucent. Add mushrooms, onion, celery, carrots, garlic, and thyme. Sauté until vegetables are fork tender, about 3–4 minutes. Add the remainder of the ingredients and bring to a boil. Reduce heat and simmer for 15–20 minutes.

Makes 6 servings

Recipe courtesy of Marlisa Brown, RD and Constance Brown-Riggs, RD, aka "Soul Sisters Cook." This recipe puts a new spin on black eyed peas.

Nutrition Facts

Serving Size 1 cup (271g)
Servings Per Container 6

Amount Per Serving

Calories 120   Calories from Fat 30

% Daily Value*

Total Fat 3.5g	**5%**
Saturated Fat 0.5g	**3%**
Trans Fat 0g	
Cholesterol 10mg	**3%**
Sodium 450mg	**19%**
Total Carbohydrate 17g	**6%**
Dietary Fiber 4g	**16%**
Sugars 3g	
Protein 6g	

Vitamin A 40% • Vitamin C 8%

Calcium 2% • Iron 8%

*Percent Daily Values are based on a 2,000 calorie diet. Your daily values may be higher or lower depending on your calorie needs:

		Calories:	2,000	2,500
Total Fat	Less than		65g	80g
Saturated Fat	Less than		20g	25g
Cholesterol	Less than		300mg	300mg
Sodium	Less than		2,400mg	2,400mg
Total Carbohydrate			300g	375g
Dietary Fiber			25g	30g

Calories per gram:
Fat 9 • Carbohydrate 4 • Protein 4

West Indian Plantain Cakes

3 medium ripe plantains
1/2 tsp. baking powder
2 Tbsp. canola oil
1/2 Tbsp. Splenda

Bring a large pan of water to boil.

Cut the ends off the plantains. Place the plantains in the water and cook until they are soft. Then drain and when they are cool enough to handle, peel the plantains, mash them well with a fork, and mix in the baking powder and sugar.

Next shape the mixture into 8 small cakes and heat the vegetable oil in a heavy frying pan and fry (over medium-low heat) the cakes on both sides until golden.

Makes 8 servings

Recipe provided by Josué Merced-Reyes, food, wine, and beverage consultant and producer and host of the Caribbean syndicated radio series *Pleasures in the Caribbean* and Buen Vivir recipes.

Nutrition Facts	
Serving Size 1 cake (95g)	
Servings Per Container 6	

Amount Per Serving	
Calories 150	Calories from Fat 45

	% Daily Value*
Total Fat 5g	8%
Saturated Fat 0g	0%
Trans Fat 0g	
Cholesterol 0mg	0%
Sodium 50mg	2%
Total Carbohydrate 29g	10%
Dietary Fiber 2g	8%
Sugars 13g	
Protein 1g	

Vitamin A 20%	•	Vitamin C 25%
Calcium 2%	•	Iron 2%

*Percent Daily Values are based on a 2,000 calorie diet. Your daily values may be higher or lower depending on your calorie needs:

		Calories:	2,000	2,500
Total Fat	Less than		65g	80g
Saturated Fat	Less than		20g	25g
Cholesterol	Less than		300mg	300mg
Sodium	Less than		2,400mg	2,400mg
Total Carbohydrate			300g	375g
Dietary Fiber			25g	30g

Calories per gram:
Fat 9 • Carbohydrate 4 • Protein 4

Haitian Pickliz

2 cups of cabbage (1/2 cabbage head)
1 medium size carrot, peeled and
    shredded
1/3 cup green beans (French cut)
1 shallot onion
8 habanero or Scotch bonnet peppers
    (see note)
1/3 cup of frozen peas (optional)
2 cups of distilled white vinegar
1/2 tsp. of salt

Sterilize a half-gallon jar and lid in hot water for 10 minutes. Let dry completely before pickling.

Put cabbage, carrot, green beans, shallot, peppers, and peas into the jar.

Pour the vinegar into the jar, add salt, and tightly screw on the lid. Shake jar to mix ingredients well.

Refrigerate for 24 hours before serving. Refrigerated pickliz will last 2 months.

Makes 10 servings

Recipe courtesy of Fabienne Volel, RD.

Nutrition Facts

Serving Size 2 Tablespoons (93g)
Servings Per Container 10

Amount Per Serving

Calories 20   Calories from Fat 0

% Daily Value*

Total Fat 0g	0%
Saturated Fat 0g	0%
Trans Fat 0g	
Cholesterol 0mg	0%
Sodium 200mg	8%
Total Carbohydrate 3g	1%
Dietary Fiber 1g	4%
Sugars 1g	
Protein 1g	

Vitamin A 15% • Vitamin C 20%

Calcium 2% • Iron 2%

*Percent Daily Values are based on a 2,000 calorie diet. Your daily values may be higher or lower depending on your calorie needs:

		Calories:	2,000	2,500
Total Fat	Less than		65g	80g
Saturated Fat	Less than		20g	25g
Cholesterol	Less than		300mg	300mg
Sodium	Less than		2,400mg	2,400mg
Total Carbohydrate			300g	375g
Dietary Fiber			25g	30g

Calories per gram:
Fat 9 • Carbohydrate 4 • Protein 4

Creole Seasoning

2 1/2 Tbsp. paprika
2 Tbsp. salt
2 Tbsp. garlic powder
1 Tbsp. black pepper
1 Tbsp. onion powder
1 Tbsp. cayenne pepper
1 Tbsp. dried oregano
1 Tbsp. dried thyme

Mix together paprika, salt, garlic powder, black pepper, onion powder, cayenne pepper, oregano, and thyme.

Mix well and keep in a sealed jar.

Makes 34 servings

Nutrition Facts

Serving Size 1 teaspoon (1.8g)
Servings Per Container 34

Amount Per Serving

Calories 5	Calories from Fat 0

	% Daily Value*
Total Fat 0g	**0%**
Saturated Fat 0g	**0%**
Trans Fat 0g	
Cholesterol 0mg	**0%**
Sodium 0mg	**0%**
Total Carbohydrate 1g	**0%**
Dietary Fiber 1g	**4%**
Sugars 0g	
Protein 0g	

Vitamin A 6%	•	Vitamin C 2%
Calcium 0%	•	Iron 2%

*Percent Daily Values are based on a 2,000 calorie diet. Your daily values may be higher or lower depending on your calorie needs:

		Calories:	2,000	2,500
Total Fat	Less than		65g	80g
Saturated Fat	Less than		20g	25g
Cholesterol	Less than		300mg	300mg
Sodium	Less than		2,400mg	2,400mg
Total Carbohydrate			300g	375g
Dietary Fiber			25g	30g

Calories per gram:
Fat 9 • Carbohydrate 4 • Protein 4

Nutrition Facts

Serving Size 1 teaspoon (3g)
Servings Per Container 34

Amount Per Serving

Calories 5	Calories from Fat 0

	% Daily Value*
Total Fat 0g	**0%**
Saturated Fat 0g	**0%**
Trans Fat 0g	
Cholesterol 0mg	**0%**
Sodium 410mg	**17%**
Total Carbohydrate 1g	**0%**
Dietary Fiber 1g	**4%**
Sugars 0g	
Protein 0g	

Vitamin A 6%	•	Vitamin C 2%
Calcium 0%	•	Iron 2%

*Percent Daily Values are based on a 2,000 calorie diet. Your daily values may be higher or lower depending on your calorie needs:

		Calories:	2,000	2,500
Total Fat	Less than		65g	80g
Saturated Fat	Less than		20g	25g
Cholesterol	Less than		300mg	300mg
Sodium	Less than		2,400mg	2,400mg
Total Carbohydrate			300g	375g
Dietary Fiber			25g	30g

Calories per gram:
Fat 9 • Carbohydrate 4 • Protein 4

For a low sodium option, cut salt down to 1 Tbsp.

Recipe provided by Josué Merced-Reyes, food, wine, and beverage consultant and producer and host of the Caribbean syndicated radio series *Pleasures in the Caribbean* and Buen Vivir recipes.

Josué suggests using this Creole seasoning on meat, chicken, seafood, or make your rice and stews with this mixture whenever your taste buds want a rich and spicy flavor.

Haitian Black Bean Sauce (Sauce pois)

1 bag (16 oz.) dry black beans
8 cups of water
4 whole cloves
2 Tbsp. vegetable or olive oil
2 scallions
5 sprigs of parsley (chopped)
1 habanero pepper
5 to 8 sprigs of thyme
1 Tbsp. salt (optional)

To cut down on cooking time, soak beans overnight.

Add black beans and water together and let boil for about 2 hours or until beans are very tender and skin is broken.

Add 2 more cups of water if water has evaporated to 1/2 of original amount. Then continue to cook until bean is completely cooked and soft.

Blend beans in a blender with parsley until it looks like a puree.

In another pot, add oil and scallions and sauté until starting to brown.

Then immediately add pureed beans, salt, cloves, thyme, and habanero pepper, and simmer for about 20 minutes.

Remove thyme before serving.

Serve with white rice.

Makes 12 servings

Courtesy Fabienne Volel, RD

Nutrition Facts

Serving Size 1/2 cup (207g)
Servings Per Container 12

Amount Per Serving

Calories 150	Calories from Fat 20

	% Daily Value*
Total Fat 2.5g	4%
Saturated Fat 0g	0%
Trans Fat 0g	
Cholesterol 0mg	0%
Sodium 200mg	8%
Total Carbohydrate 24g	8%
Dietary Fiber 3g	12%
Sugars 3g	
Protein 8g	

Vitamin A 2%	•	Vitamin C 10%
Calcium 0%	•	Iron 10%

*Percent Daily Values are based on a 2,000 calorie diet. Your daily values may be higher or lower depending on your calorie needs:

	Calories:	2,000	2,500
Total Fat	Less than	65g	80g
Saturated Fat	Less than	20g	25g
Cholesterol	Less than	300mg	300mg
Sodium	Less than	2,400mg	2,400mg
Total Carbohydrate		300g	375g
Dietary Fiber		25g	30g

Calories per gram:
Fat 9 • Carbohydrate 4 • Protein 4

Main Dishes

Mango Pork

2 mangos, peeled
12 ounces pork tenderloin
Cooking spray
Pinch salt
Pinch black pepper
Hot pepper sauce (to taste)

Put the pulp of 1 mango in food processor or blender.

Take a second mango and cut into small cubes.

Quickly brown 1-inch thick pork medallions over medium-high heat in a skillet sprayed with cooking spray. Season with salt and pepper. Reduce heat and cook for another 5 minutes. Remove to a plate.

Add the mango puree to the skillet and cook puree, scraping up brown bits of pork, for about 30 seconds. Add dash hot sauce and the mango cubes, heating through. Spoon sauce over pork and serve.

Makes 2 ½ servings

Nutrition Facts	
Serving Size 4 oz (303g)	
Servings Per Container 2 1/2	
Amount Per Serving	
Calories 260	Calories from Fat 35
	% Daily Value*
Total Fat 4g	**6%**
Saturated Fat 1g	**5%**
Trans Fat 0g	
Cholesterol 90mg	**30%**
Sodium 135mg	**6%**
Total Carbohydrate 27g	**9%**
Dietary Fiber 2g	**8%**
Sugars 2g	
Protein 29g	
Vitamin A 60% • Vitamin C 25%	
Calcium 0% • Iron 8%	

*Percent Daily Values are based on a 2,000 calorie diet. Your daily values may be higher or lower depending on your calorie needs:

		Calories:	2,000	2,500
Total Fat	Less than		65g	80g
Saturated Fat	Less than		20g	25g
Cholesterol	Less than		300mg	300mg
Sodium	Less than		2,400mg	2,400mg
Total Carbohydrate			300g	375g
Dietary Fiber			25g	30g

Calories per gram:
Fat 9 • Carbohydrate 4 • Protein 4

Recipe provided by Josué Merced-Reyes, food, wine, and beverage consultant and producer and host of the Caribbean syndicated radio series *Pleasures in the Caribbean* and Buen Vivir recipes.

Haitian Legume

2 lbs. of round steak, trimmed of all fat
    and cut into 2-inch cubes
2 limes, juiced
3 Tbsp. of tomato paste
1/3 cup of vegetable oil
2 cups of water
1 eggplant, cubed
2 chayotes
1 red bell pepper
3 scallions, chopped fine
2 garlic clove, minced
A bunch of fresh parsley, chopped
4 sprigs of thyme (optional)
1 habanero pepper
20 oz. of frozen ford hook lima beans
2 cups of fresh spinach, or frozen
    spinach
3 carrots peeled and cubed
1 Tbsp. of salt or salt to taste
1 Maggi cube (chicken flavor bouillon)
    (optional)
2 Tbsp. of pickliz (optional)

Nutrition Facts		
Serving Size 1 cup (344g)		
Servings Per Container 10		
Amount Per Serving		
Calories 350	Calories from Fat 120	
		% Daily Value*
Total Fat 14g		22%
Saturated Fat 3g		15%
Trans Fat 0g		
Cholesterol 75mg		25%
Sodium 350mg		15%
Total Carbohydrate 22g		7%
Dietary Fiber 7g		28%
Sugars 6g		
Protein 37g		
Vitamin A 50%	•	Vitamin C 70%
Calcium 6%	•	Iron 25%

*Percent Daily Values are based on a 2,000 calorie diet. Your daily values may be higher or lower depending on your calorie needs:

		Calories:	2,000	2,500
Total Fat	Less than		65g	80g
Saturated Fat	Less than		20g	25g
Cholesterol	Less than		300mg	300mg
Sodium	Less than		2,400mg	2,400mg
Total Carbohydrate			300g	375g
Dietary Fiber			25g	30g

Calories per gram:
    Fat 9 • Carbohydrate 4 • Protein 4

Wash beef with lime juice and allow to marinate for 10 minutes. Rinse with cold water.

In large pot, add oil, and when oil is hot add scallions and garlic and cook for 1 minute and then add tomato paste. Stir the scallions, garlic, and tomato paste for about 1 more minute, until mildly brown. Add beef, water, red bell pepper, thyme, parsley, and salt. Add habanero pepper whole; do not let it open or else food will be very spicy.

In a separate pot, steam eggplant and chayote until very tender. Mash them together. When meat is tender, remove habanero pepper. Add lima beans and carrots. When carrots are tender add mashed eggplant and chayote. Add spinach and the Maggi cube if desired.

Add thyme for about 5 minutes and remove before serving. Salt to taste.

Makes 10 servings

Recipe courtesy of Fabienne Volel, RD.

Cornmeal Crusted Catfish

1/4 cup crushed pecans
1 tsp. paprika
1 1/2 tsp. garlic powder
2 tsp. minced onions
1/2 tsp. black pepper
1/2 tsp. salt
3 Tbsp. low-fat mayonnaise
2 Tbsp. apricot preserves
1 lb. catfish fillets
Cooking spray

In small bowl, mix together cornmeal, pecans, paprika, garlic powder, onion, pepper, and salt.

Heat medium nonstick skillet over medium heat until hot.

Pour in cornmeal mixture. Cook and stir about 3 minutes or until cornmeal begins to brown. Transfer to platter and set aside.

Nutrition Facts		
Serving Size 4 ounces (154g)		
Servings Per Container 4		
Amount Per Serving		
Calories 270	Calories from Fat 130	
		% Daily Value*
Total Fat 14g		22%
Saturated Fat 2.5g		13%
Trans Fat 0g		
Cholesterol 55mg		18%
Sodium 450mg		19%
Total Carbohydrate 17g		6%
Dietary Fiber 2g		8%
Sugars 8g		
Protein 19g		
Vitamin A 8%	•	Vitamin C 2%
Calcium 2%	•	Iron 8%

*Percent Daily Values are based on a 2,000 calorie diet. Your daily values may be higher or lower depending on your calorie needs:

	Calories:	2,000	2,500
Total Fat	Less than	65g	80g
Saturated Fat	Less than	20g	25g
Cholesterol	Less than	300mg	300mg
Sodium	Less than	2,400mg	2,400mg
Total Carbohydrate		300g	375g
Dietary Fiber		25g	30g

Calories per gram:
Fat 9 • Carbohydrate 4 • Protein 4

In small bowl or cup, mix together mayonnaise and preserves. Brush on both sides of catfish fillets. Dredge fillets in toasted cornmeal mixture.

Coat medium skillet with nonstick cooking spray and heat until hot. Reduce to medium heat. Add fillets. Cook until browned.

Carefully turn and brown other side until cooked through.

Makes 4 servings

Recipe courtesy of Marlisa Brown, RD, and Constance Brown-Riggs, RD, aka "Soul Sisters Cook." The cornmeal and pecans add a little crunch to this delicate, tender fish.

Cumin Roast Goat

1 cup chopped onions
6 garlic cloves, minced
3 Tbsp. cumin
1 Tbsp. coriander
3 lbs. goat, shoulder or leg bone-in roast

Mash together chopped onions, garlic cloves, cumin, and coriander to form a paste. Pierce a goat shoulder roast all over and rub the paste into the meat. Marinate overnight.

Preheat the oven to 400°F.

Sear the meat loosely covered with foil in a roasting pan at 400°F for 15 minutes. Then reduce to 350°F and roast for another two hours (depending on weight). Remove the foil for the last 15 minutes of cooking. Let roast rest 10 minutes before carving.

Makes 8 servings

Recipe provided by Josué Merced-Reyes, food, wine, and beverage consultant and producer and host of the Caribbean syndicated radio series *Pleasures in the Caribbean* and Buen Vivir recipes.

Nutrition Facts

Serving Size 4 1/2 oz (173g)
Servings Per Container 9

Amount Per Serving

Calories 180   Calories from Fat 35

	% Daily Value*
Total Fat 4g	**6%**
Saturated Fat 1g	**5%**
Trans Fat 0g	
Cholesterol 85mg	**28%**
Sodium 130mg	**5%**
Total Carbohydrate 3g	**1%**
Dietary Fiber 1g	**4%**
Sugars 1g	
Protein 32g	

Vitamin A 0%	•	Vitamin C 4%
Calcium 4%	•	Iron 30%

*Percent Daily Values are based on a 2,000 calorie diet. Your daily values may be higher or lower depending on your calorie needs:

	Calories:	2,000	2,500
Total Fat	Less than	65g	80g
Saturated Fat	Less than	20g	25g
Cholesterol	Less than	300mg	300mg
Sodium	Less than	2,400mg	2,400mg
Total Carbohydrate		300g	375g
Dietary Fiber		25g	30g

Calories per gram:
   Fat 9 • Carbohydrate 4 • Protein 4

Home-style Meat Loaf

1/2 lb. ground beef, extra lean
1/2 lb. ground veal
1/2 lb. ground pork
1/4 cup tomato paste
1/4 cup onion, chopped
1/4 cup green peppers
1/2 cup tomatoes, fresh, blanched,
    chopped
1/4 tsp. ground black pepper
1 tsp. fresh chili pepper
2 tsp. orange rind, grated
1 tsp. thyme, crushed
1/4 cup bread crumbs, finely grated
2 egg whites, beaten

Preheat oven to 350°F.

In a large bowl mix all ingredients together.

Place mixture in a 1-pound loaf pan. Wet fingertips with water and smooth off the top of mixture.

Cover and bake for 50 minutes. Uncover and continue baking for 15 minutes.

Makes 5 servings

Recipe courtesy of Lawrence Riggs, RD.

Nutrition Facts

Serving Size 5 1/2 oz (170g)
Servings Per Container 6

Amount Per Serving

Calories 220   Calories from Fat 100

% Daily Value*

Total Fat 11g	**17%**
Saturated Fat 4g	**20%**
Trans Fat 0g	
Cholesterol 75mg	**25%**
Sodium 140mg	**6%**
Total Carbohydrate 7g	**2%**
Dietary Fiber 1g	**4%**
Sugars 2g	
Protein 23g	

Vitamin A 6%	•	Vitamin C 20%
Calcium 2%	•	Iron 10%

*Percent Daily Values are based on a 2,000 calorie diet. Your daily values may be higher or lower depending on your calorie needs:

		Calories:	2,000	2,500
Total Fat	Less than		65g	80g
Saturated Fat	Less than		20g	25g
Cholesterol	Less than		300mg	300mg
Sodium	Less than		2,400mg	2,400mg
Total Carbohydrate			300g	375g
Dietary Fiber			25g	30g

Calories per gram:
  Fat 9 • Carbohydrate 4 • Protein 4

Oven Fried Fish

2 lb. fish fillets—any fish you enjoy

1 Tbsp. lemon juice, fresh

1/4 cup fat-free or 1% buttermilk

2 drops hot sauce

1 tsp. fresh garlic, minced

1/4 tsp. white pepper, ground

1/4 tsp. salt

1/4 tsp. onion powder

1/2 cup cornflakes, crumbled or regular bread crumbs

1 Tbsp. vegetable oil

1 fresh lemon cut in wedges

Preheat oven to 475°F.

Clean and rinse fish. Wipe fillets with lemon juice and pat dry.

Combine milk, hot sauce, and garlic.

Combine pepper, salt, and onion powder with crumbs and place on plate.

Let fillets sit briefly in milk. Remove and coat fillets on both sides with seasoned crumbs. Let stand briefly until coating sticks to each side of fish. Arrange on lightly oiled, shallow baking dish.

Bake for 20 minutes on middle rack without turning.

Cut into 6 pieces. Serve with fresh lemon.

Nutrition Facts		
Serving Size (197g)		
Servings Per Container		
Amount Per Serving		
Calories 210	Calories from Fat 45	
		% Daily Value*
Total Fat 5g		**8%**
Saturated Fat 1g		**5%**
Trans Fat 0g		
Cholesterol 75mg		**25%**
Sodium 310mg		**13%**
Total Carbohydrate 9g		**3%**
Dietary Fiber 1g		**4%**
Sugars 2g		
Protein 31g		
Vitamin A 2%	•	Vitamin C 15%
Calcium 8%	•	Iron 6%

*Percent Daily Values are based on a 2,000 calorie diet. Your daily values may be higher or lower depending on your calorie needs:

	Calories:	2,000	2,500
Total Fat	Less than	65g	80g
Saturated Fat	Less than	20g	25g
Cholesterol	Less than	300mg	300mg
Sodium	Less than	2,400mg	2,400mg
Total Carbohydrate		300g	375g
Dietary Fiber		25g	30g

Calories per gram:
Fat 9 • Carbohydrate 4 • Protein 4

Makes 6 servings

Recipe from National Institute of Health, Heart Healthy Home Cooking.

Easy Rice and Beans

1 can of red kidney beans (no sodium
  added)
1 cup of brown rice
1 4-oz. can of low-sodium tomato sauce
1 tsp. of oregano
2 cloves of garlic
1 tsp. of black pepper
1 tsp. of olive, canola, or vegetable oil
1 onion
1 green, red, or yellow pepper
2 cloves of garlic
sprinkle of salt
1 cup of water

Dice the onions, garlic, and pepper.

Cook the rice according to the directions
on the package. Add a teaspoon of olive,
canola, or vegetable oil (and a sprinkle
of salt) to the same pot and stir.

Drain and rinse the beans and add them
to the pot of rice once the rice is almost
done cooking.

Add a cup of water and the tomato
sauce to the pot. Add the diced onions,
garlic, pepper, and spices/herbs.

Heat for about 10 more minutes (or
until done) and serve.

Nutrition Facts	
Serving Size 1 cup (253g)	
Servings Per Container 5	
Amount Per Serving	
Calories 230	Calories from Fat 20
	% Daily Value*
Total Fat 2.5g	**4%**
Saturated Fat 0g	**0%**
Trans Fat 0g	
Cholesterol 0mg	**0%**
Sodium 25mg	**1%**
Total Carbohydrate 47g	**16%**
Dietary Fiber 9g	**36%**
Sugars 4g	
Protein 10g	
Vitamin A 4% • Vitamin C 45%	
Calcium 6% • Iron 10%	

*Percent Daily Values are based on a 2,000 calorie
diet. Your daily values may be higher or lower
depending on your calorie needs:

	Calories:	2,000	2,500
Total Fat	Less than	65g	80g
Saturated Fat	Less than	20g	25g
Cholesterol	Less than	300mg	300mg
Sodium	Less than	2,400mg	2,400mg
Total Carbohydrate		300g	375g
Dietary Fiber		25g	30g

Calories per gram:
Fat 9 • Carbohydrate 4 • Protein 4

Makes 5 servings

When you're strapped for cash and time, this recipe comes in handy. Courtesy
Jessica Jones, freelance writer.

Escoveitch Fish

2 lbs. fish (snapper, jacks, sprats, parrot, grunt, or kingfish)*
Juice of 2 limes
Pinch of salt
Pinch of black pepper
1 Tbsp. canola oil
2 onions sliced
2 hot peppers sliced, like Scotch Bonnet
2 Tbsp. pimento berries
1 cup distilled vinegar

*Any fish can be used.

Nutrition Facts		
Serving Size 4 oz (266g)		
Servings Per Container 6		
Amount Per Serving		
Calories 220	Calories from Fat 50	
		% Daily Value*
Total Fat 6g		**9%**
Saturated Fat 1g		5%
Trans Fat 0g		
Cholesterol 80mg		**27%**
Sodium 300mg		**13%**
Total Carbohydrate 8g		**3%**
Dietary Fiber 1g		4%
Sugars 3g		
Protein 32g		
Vitamin A 25%	•	Vitamin C 20%
Calcium 8%	•	Iron 15%

*Percent Daily Values are based on a 2,000 calorie diet. Your daily values may be higher or lower depending on your calorie needs:

		Calories:	2,000	2,500
Total Fat	Less than		65g	80g
Saturated Fat	Less than		20g	25g
Cholesterol	Less than		300mg	300mg
Sodium	Less than		2,400mg	2,400mg
Total Carbohydrate			300g	375g
Dietary Fiber			25g	30g

Calories per gram:
Fat 9 • Carbohydrate 4 • Protein 4

Clean and wash the fish, rub fish with lime juice, and dry with paper towels.

Sprinkle fish on both sides and inside with salt and pepper.

Heat oil in a frying pan until it is very hot and begins to smoke very slightly. Place the fish in the hot oil one at a time, taking care that they do not overlap.

Reduce the heat a little and fry the fish on both sides. (If they are difficult to turn, the oil was not hot enough. Leave them for a couple of minutes to allow the underside to brown, and then turn.)

When the fish are done, drain, pat off excess oil with a paper towel, and arrange them on a large platter or in a deep bowl.

Put in the same frying pan the onions, hot peppers, pimento, vinegar and a little salt to taste. Bring the mixture to a boil and simmer for about 2 minutes. The onions should remain crunchy.

Remove onion mixture from the heat; pour this hot pickle over the fish. Serve hot or cold.

Makes 6 servings

This recipe is complements of Leslene Gordon, PhD, RD. Escoveitch fish is usually prepared with snapper, jacks, sprats, parrot, grunt, or kingfish. Escoveitch fish is traditionally served with bammy (a cassava product), hard-dough bread, festival (similar to hush puppies), or Johnny cakes.

Old Fashion Beef Stew

2 cups cubed beef
1/2 cup celery
1/2 cup Spanish onion
1 cup red bliss potato
1/2 cup crushed plum tomato
4 tsp. fresh thyme
4 tsp. fresh parsley
4 tsp. fresh rosemary
1/2 cup frozen peas
1 cup red wine
4 cup low sodium beef stock
4 Tbsp. olive oil
3 Tbsp. cornstarch
1/3 cup water
1/4 cup carrots
Salt and pepper to taste

Nutrition Facts	
Serving Size 1 cup (307g)	
Servings Per Container 8	
Amount Per Serving	
Calories 330 Calories from Fat 120	
	% Daily Value*
Total Fat 13g	**20%**
Saturated Fat 3.5g	**18%**
Trans Fat 0g	
Cholesterol 70mg	**23%**
Sodium 140mg	**6%**
Total Carbohydrate 12g	**4%**
Dietary Fiber 2g	**8%**
Sugars 3g	
Protein 33g	
Vitamin A 25% • Vitamin C 25%	
Calcium 4% • Iron 20%	

*Percent Daily Values are based on a 2,000 calorie diet. Your daily values may be higher or lower depending on your calorie needs:

		Calories:	2,000	2,500
Total Fat	Less than		65g	80g
Saturated Fat	Less than		20g	25g
Cholesterol	Less than		300mg	300mg
Sodium	Less than		2,400mg	2,400mg
Total Carbohydrate			300g	375g
Dietary Fiber			25g	30g

Calories per gram:
Fat 9 • Carbohydrate 4 • Protein 4

Heat oil in large stock pot over medium heat. Add beef and brown on all sides, stirring occasionally. When brown, remove from pot and reserve.

In same pot (don't clean) add onions and cook for 4 minutes to caramelize the onions, then add celery, parsley, carrots, and thyme and sauté for 5 minutes until tender.

Deglaze vegetables with red wine and let simmer until the liquid is reduced by 1/2. Add beef stock, beef, and tomato. Bring to a boil, add potatoes, and simmer.

Mix cornstarch and water to create slurry and add to stew and continue to simmer 15 to 20 minutes until potatoes are tender. Fold in peas and simmer an additional 5 minutes.

Makes 8 servings

Courtesy Chef Marc Anthony Bynum.

Turkey Burger

1/2 cup diced onion
2 Tbsp. olive oil
2 lbs. lean ground turkey meat
1 large egg
1/2 tsp. black pepper
1/4 tsp. salt
3 tsp. basil, chopped
1 Tbsp. tomato paste
1/4 cup grated parmesan cheese, reduced
    fat
Non stick cooking spray

Dice a small onion. In a small pan, heat oil and add onions.

Sauté for 5 minutes until golden brown, stirring occasionally. Drain onto paper towel to drain excess oil and water. Reserve.

In a large mixing bowl, add ground turkey, egg, onion, pepper, salt, basil, tomato paste, and parmesan cheese. Mix all ingredients until fully incorporated. Shape mixture into 6 patties.

Heat a nonstick skillet over medium heat until hot. Place burgers in skillet and cook four minutes on each side. Remove from heat and serve.

Nutrition Facts

Serving Size 5 oz (173g)
Servings Per Container 6

Amount Per Serving

Calories 190   Calories from Fat 30

% Daily Value*

Total Fat 3.5g	5%
Saturated Fat 0.5g	3%
Trans Fat 0g	
Cholesterol 100mg	33%
Sodium 250mg	10%
Total Carbohydrate 1g	0%
Dietary Fiber 0g	0%
Sugars 1g	
Protein 39g	

Vitamin A 2%	•	Vitamin C 2%
Calcium 4%	•	Iron 10%

*Percent Daily Values are based on a 2,000 calorie diet. Your daily values may be higher or lower depending on your calorie needs:

		Calories:	2,000	2,500
Total Fat	Less than		65g	80g
Saturated Fat	Less than		20g	25g
Cholesterol	Less than		300mg	300mg
Sodium	Less than		2,400mg	2,400mg
Total Carbohydrate			300g	375g
Dietary Fiber			25g	30g

Calories per gram:
    Fat 9 • Carbohydrate 4 • Protein 4

Makes 6 servings

Recipe courtesy of Chef Marc Anthony Bynum.

Caribbean Chili and Sweet Potatoes

1 medium sweet potato
1 15-ounce can low-sodium black
   beans
2 minced jalapeno peppers
2 diced tomatoes
Salt to taste

Preheat oven to 350ºF

Bake sweet potato.

Meanwhile, combine black beans, jalapeño chilies, and diced tomatoes. Cook over low heat for 30 minutes. Check for seasoning.

Cut the sweet potato into four pieces. Cover each quarter with the 1/2 cup black bean mixture and serve.

Makes 4 servings

Recipe provided by Josué Merced-Reyes, food, wine, and beverage consultant and producer and host of the Caribbean syndicated radio series *Pleasures in the Caribbean* and Buen Vivir recipes.

Nutrition Facts

Serving Size 1/2 cup bean mixture &
1/4 potato (206g)
Servings Per Container 4

Amount Per Serving

Calories 130   Calories from Fat 5

% Daily Value*

Total Fat 0.5g	**1%**
Saturated Fat 0g	**0%**
Trans Fat 0g	
Cholesterol 0mg	**0%**
Sodium 440mg	**18%**
Total Carbohydrate 26g	**9%**
Dietary Fiber 7g	**28%**
Sugars 5g	
Protein 7g	

Vitamin A 120% • Vitamin C 35%

Calcium 6% • Iron 10%

*Percent Daily Values are based on a 2,000 calorie diet. Your daily values may be higher or lower depending on your calorie needs:

		Calories:	2,000	2,500
Total Fat	Less than		65g	80g
Saturated Fat	Less than		20g	25g
Cholesterol	Less than		300mg	300mg
Sodium	Less than		2,400mg	2,400mg
Total Carbohydrate			300g	375g
Dietary Fiber			25g	30g

Calories per gram:
   Fat 9 • Carbohydrate 4 • Protein 4

Lawrence's Cajun Style Gumbo

1 Tbsp. vegetable oil
1/4 cup all purpose flour
3 cups low sodium, low fat chicken broth
1 lb. chicken breast, skinless and boneless
    cut into 1/2-inch pieces
1/2 cup yellow onion
1/4 cup celery chopped
4 cloves garlic minced
2 scallions chopped
1 whole bay leaf
2 tsp. thyme, ground
2 tsp. jalapeno pepper
1 tsp. crushed red pepper
1 tsp. poultry seasoning
2 tsp. gumbo file
2 tsp. gravy master
1/2 cup okra

Nutrition Facts
Serving Size 3/4 cup (206g)
Servings Per Container 8

Amount Per Serving	
Calories 170	Calories from Fat 70

	% Daily Value*
Total Fat 8g	**12%**
Saturated Fat 2g	**10%**
Trans Fat 0g	
Cholesterol 55mg	**18%**
Sodium 240mg	**10%**
Total Carbohydrate 6g	**2%**
Dietary Fiber 1g	**4%**
Sugars 1g	
Protein 18g	

Vitamin A 4%	•	Vitamin C 6%
Calcium 4%	•	Iron 8%

*Percent Daily Values are based on a 2,000 calorie diet. Your daily values may be higher or lower depending on your calorie needs:

	Calories:	2,000	2,500
Total Fat	Less than	65g	80g
Saturated Fat	Less than	20g	25g
Cholesterol	Less than	300mg	300mg
Sodium	Less than	2,400mg	2,400mg
Total Carbohydrate		300g	375g
Dietary Fiber		25g	30g

Calories per gram:
Fat 9 • Carbohydrate 4 • Protein 4

Preheat oven to 400°F.

Add oil to small pot, stir in flour.

Place in oven, stirring constantly until flour begins to turn golden brown.

Take pot out of oven and continue preparation on top of the stove.

Slowly stir in broth using wire whisk and cook for 2 minutes.

Add all ingredients except okra. Bring to boil, then reduce heat and let simmer for 45 minutes.

Add okra and let cook for 15 to 20 additional minutes.

Remove bay leaf.

Serve hot in bowl alone or over rice.

Makes 8 servings

Courtesy Lawrence Riggs, RD.

Crispy Oven-Fried Chicken

1/2 cup fat free milk or buttermilk
1 tsp. poultry seasoning
1 cup cornflakes, crumbled
1 1/2 Tbsp. onion powder
1 1/2 Tbsp. garlic powder
2 tsp. black pepper
2 tsp. dried hot pepper, crushed
1 tsp. ginger, ground
8 pieces chicken, skinless (4 breast, 4
    drumsticks)
A few shakes paprika
1 tsp. vegetable oil

Preheat oven to 350°F.

Add 1/2 tsp. of poultry seasoning to milk

Combine all other spices with cornflake crumbs, and place in plastic bag

Wash chicken and pat dry. Dip chicken into milk and shake to remove excess. Quickly shake in bag with seasonings and crumbs, and remove the chicken from the bag.

Refrigerate chicken for 1 hour.

Remove chicken from refrigerator and sprinkle lightly with paprika for color.

Space chicken evenly on greased baking pan. Cover with aluminum foil and bake for 40 minutes. Remove foil and continue baking for another 30 to 40 minutes or until meat can easily be pulled away from the bone with fork. Drumsticks may require less baking time than breasts. Crumbs will form crispy "skin."

Note: Do not turn chicken during baking.

Makes 10 servings

Recipe from National Institute of Health, Heart Healthy Home Cooking

---

Nutrition Facts

Serving Size 1/2 breast or 2 small drumstricks (83g)
Servings Per Container 10

Amount Per Serving

Calories 140   Calories from Fat 45

% Daily Value*

	% Daily Value*
Total Fat 5g	8%
Saturated Fat 1.5g	8%
Trans Fat 0g	
Cholesterol 55mg	18%
Sodium 85mg	4%
Total Carbohydrate 6g	2%
Dietary Fiber 1g	4%
Sugars 1g	
Protein 18g	

Vitamin A 6%   •   Vitamin C 6%

Calcium 4%   •   Iron 8%

*Percent Daily Values are based on a 2,000 calorie diet. Your daily values may be higher or lower depending on your calorie needs:

	Calories:	2,000	2,500
Total Fat	Less than	65g	80g
Saturated Fat	Less than	20g	25g
Cholesterol	Less than	300mg	300mg
Sodium	Less than	2,400mg	2,400mg
Total Carbohydrate		300g	375g
Dietary Fiber		25g	30g

Calories per gram:
    Fat 9 • Carbohydrate 4 • Protein 4

Sweets

Upside Down Pineapple Cake

1 20-oz. can sliced pineapple in juice
1 Tbsp. molasses
1/2 tsp. ground cinnamon
1/4 cup margarine
1/2 tsp. vanilla extract
1 cup brown sugar, Splenda blend
2 egg whites
1 1/2 cup flour
1/2 tsp. baking soda

Heat oven to 350°F.

Spray 9-inch Teflon pan with cooking spray.

Put pineapple on the bottom of the pan (reserve pineapple juice). Cover with molasses and cinnamon.

Mix together margarine, Splenda, and egg whites. Add 3/4 cup pineapple juice and flour and blend until smooth.

Bake for 30 to 35 minutes.

Makes 12 servings

Recipe courtesy Marlisa Brown, RD, and Constance Brown-Riggs, RD, aka "Soul Sisters Cook."

Nutrition Facts

Serving Size 1 slice (67g)
Servings Per Container 12

Amount Per Serving

Calories 130   Calories from Fat 35

	% Daily Value*
Total Fat 3.5g	5%
Saturated Fat 0.5g	3%
Trans Fat 0.5g	
Cholesterol 0mg	0%
Sodium 100mg	4%
Total Carbohydrate 21g	7%
Dietary Fiber 1g	4%
Sugars 8g	
Protein 2g	

Vitamin A 4% • Vitamin C 6%

Calcium 2% • Iron 4%

*Percent Daily Values are based on a 2,000 calorie diet. Your daily values may be higher or lower depending on your calorie needs:

	Calories:	2,000	2,500
Total Fat	Less than	65g	80g
Saturated Fat	Less than	20g	25g
Cholesterol	Less than	300mg	300mg
Sodium	Less than	2,400mg	2,400mg
Total Carbohydrate		300g	375g
Dietary Fiber		25g	30g

Calories per gram:
Fat 9 • Carbohydrate 4 • Protein 4

Southern Banana Pudding

3 3/4 cups cold, fat-free milk

2 small packages (4 serving size) of fat-free, sugar-free, instant vanilla pudding and pie-filling mix

32 reduced-fat vanilla wafers

2 medium bananas, sliced

2 cups fat-free, frozen whipped topping, thawed

Nutrition Facts	
Serving Size 3/4 cup (152g)	
Servings Per Container 10	
Amount Per Serving	
Calories 150	Calories from Fat 0
	% Daily Value*
Total Fat 0g	**0%**
Saturated Fat 0g	**0%**
Trans Fat 0g	
Cholesterol 0mg	**0%**
Sodium 210mg	**9%**
Total Carbohydrate 33g	**11%**
Dietary Fiber 1g	**4%**
Sugars 16g	
Protein 4g	
Vitamin A 4% • Vitamin C 4%	
Calcium 10% • Iron 2%	

*Percent Daily Values are based on a 2,000 calorie diet. Your daily values may be higher or lower depending on your calorie needs:

		Calories:	2,000	2,500
Total Fat	Less than		65g	80g
Saturated Fat	Less than		20g	25g
Cholesterol	Less than		300mg	300mg
Sodium	Less than		2,400mg	2,400mg
Total Carbohydrate			300g	375g
Dietary Fiber			25g	30g

Calories per gram:
Fat 9 • Carbohydrate 4 • Protein 4

Fat 9 • Carbohydrate 4 • Protein 4

Mix 3 1/2 cups of the milk with the pudding mixes. Beat the pudding mixture with a wire whisk for 2 minutes until it is well blended. Let stand for 5 minutes.

Fold 1 cup of the whipped topping into the pudding mix.

Arrange a layer of wafers on the bottom and sides of a 2-quart serving bowl. Drizzle 2 tablespoons of the remaining milk over the wafers. Add a layer of banana slices and top with one-third of the pudding.

Repeat layers, drizzling wafer layer with remaining milk and ending with pudding. Spread the remaining whipped topping over the pudding.

Refrigerate for at least 3 hours before serving.

Makes 10 servings

Recipe from National Institute of Health, Heart Healthy Home Cooking.

Summer Breeze Smoothie

1 cup yogurt, plain, nonfat
6 medium strawberries
1 cup pineapple, crushed, canned in juice
1 medium banana
1 tsp. vanilla extract
4 ice cubes

Place all ingredients in blender and puree until smooth.

Serve in frosted glass.

Makes 3 servings

Recipe from National Institute of Health, Heart Healthy Home Cooking.

Nutrition Facts

Serving Size 1 cup (245g)
Servings Per Container 3

Amount Per Serving

Calories 150 · Calories from Fat 0

% Daily Value*

Total Fat 0g	**0%**
Saturated Fat 0g	**0%**
Trans Fat 0g	
Cholesterol 0mg	**0%**
Sodium 80mg	**3%**
Total Carbohydrate 33g	**11%**
Dietary Fiber 2g	**8%**
Sugars 27g	
Protein 6g	

Vitamin A 2% · Vitamin C 60%

Calcium 15% · Iron 2%

*Percent Daily Values are based on a 2,000 calorie diet. Your daily values may be higher or lower depending on your calorie needs:

	Calories:	2,000	2,500
Total Fat	Less than	65g	80g
Saturated Fat	Less than	20g	25g
Cholesterol	Less than	300mg	300mg
Sodium	Less than	2,400mg	2,400mg
Total Carbohydrate		300g	375g
Dietary Fiber		25g	30g

Calories per gram:
Fat 9 · Carbohydrate 4 · Protein 4
Fat 9 · Carbohydrate 4 · Protein 4

Mock-Southern Sweet Potato Pie

Crust

1 1/4 cup flour
1/4 tsp. sugar
1/3 cup fat-free milk
2 Tbsp. vegetable oil

Filling

1/4 cup white sugar
1/4 cup brown sugar
1/2 tsp. salt
1/4 tsp. nutmeg
3 large eggs, beaten
1/4 cup fat-free evaporated milk
1 tsp. vanilla extract
3 cups sweet potatoes (cooked and
     mashed)

Preheat oven to 350°F.

To prepare crust:

Combine flour and sugar in bowl.

Add milk and oil to flour mixture.

Stir with fork until well mixed. Form pastry into smooth ball with hands.

Roll ball between two 12-inch squares of wax paper, using short, brisk strokes, until pastry reaches edges of paper.

Peel off top paper and invert crust into pie plate.

To prepare filling:

Combine sugars, salt, nutmeg, and eggs. Add milk and vanilla. Stir.

Add sweet potatoes and mix well. Pour mixture into pie shell.

Bake for 60 minutes or until crust is golden brown. Cool and cut into 16 slices.

Makes 16 servings

Recipe from National Institute of Health, Heart Healthy Home Cooking.

Nutrition Facts

Serving Size 1 slice (83g)
Servings Per Container 16

Amount Per Serving

Calories 130   Calories from Fat 25

	% Daily Value*
Total Fat 2.5g	**4%**
Saturated Fat 0g	**0%**
Trans Fat 0g	
Cholesterol 40mg	**13%**
Sodium 130mg	**5%**
Total Carbohydrate 24g	**8%**
Dietary Fiber 1g	**4%**
Sugars 9g	
Protein 3g	

Vitamin A 80% • Vitamin C 4%

Calcium 4% • Iron 6%

*Percent Daily Values are based on a 2,000 calorie diet. Your daily values may be higher or lower depending on your calorie needs:

	Calories:	2,000	2,500
Total Fat	Less than	65g	80g
Saturated Fat	Less than	20g	25g
Cholesterol	Less than	300mg	300mg
Sodium	Less than	2,400mg	2,400mg
Total Carbohydrate		300g	375g
Dietary Fiber		25g	30g

Calories per gram:
Fat 9 • Carbohydrate 4 • Protein 4
Fat 9 • Carbohydrate 4 • Protein 4

Tangy Fruit Salad

2 Tbsp. instant sugar-free vanilla
    pudding mix*
1 cup light vanilla yogurt
1 15-oz. can pineapple chunks, in juice,
    drained
1 11-oz. can mandarin oranges, in juice,
    drained
1 cup grapes
2 medium bananas sliced

Combine pudding mix and yogurt. Mix fruit in medium bowl.

Stir fruit into yogurt mixture

Refrigerate. Serve when chilled.

*The leftover pudding mix can be blended with milk (according to the box instructions) and used as a topping for berries.

Makes 6 servings

Recipe from National Institute of Health, Heart Healthy Home Cooking.

Nutrition Facts

Serving Size 1/2 cup (236g)
Servings Per Container 6

Amount Per Serving

Calories 140   Calories from Fat 0

	% Daily Value*
Total Fat 0g	**0%**
Saturated Fat 0g	**0%**
Trans Fat 0g	
Cholesterol 0mg	**0%**
Sodium 50mg	**2%**
Total Carbohydrate 36g	**12%**
Dietary Fiber 3g	**12%**
Sugars 28g	
Protein 3g	

Vitamin A 15% • Vitamin C 45%

Calcium 8% • Iron 2%

*Percent Daily Values are based on a 2,000 calorie diet. Your daily values may be higher or lower depending on your calorie needs:

		Calories:	2,000	2,500
Total Fat	Less than		65g	80g
Saturated Fat	Less than		20g	25g
Cholesterol	Less than		300mg	300mg
Sodium	Less than		2,400mg	2,400mg
Total Carbohydrate			300g	375g
Dietary Fiber			25g	30g

Calories per gram:
Fat 9 • Carbohydrate 4 • Protein 4

Fat 9 • Carbohydrate 4 • Protein 4

APPENDIX C

CARIBBEAN AND SOUL FOOD LIST

Appendix C provides a list of over 100 traditional foods from the American South and the Caribbean—foods that aren't easily found in most books of food counts. It doesn't have white bread or Cheerios. But you will find foods like bammy bread, akee, callaloo, crawfish, and trotters. Carbohydrate counts and nutrient information for these foods will help you successfully incorporate them in your daily meal planning.

STARCH CHOICES

	Edible Portion	Cal	Fat (g)	Sat Fat (g)	Carb (g)	Fiber (g)	Sod. (mgs)	Carb Choices	Exchanges
Breads									
Bammy	1	217	Trace	0	53.5	0	325	3 1/2	3 1/2 Starch
Corn bread, 3 ¾" × 2 ½" × ¾"	1	188	6	1.6	29	1.4	467	2	2 Starch, 1 Fat
Bread dressing/ stuffing									
Corn bread	1/2 cup	179	8.8	1.8	21.9	2.9	455	1 1/2	1 1/2 Starch, 2 Fat
Naan 8" × 2"	1/4	80	1	0	15			1	1 Starch
Hot Cereals									
Cooked Corn (Hominy) Grits									
White	1 cup	145	Trace	0.1	31	0.5	0	2	2 Starch
Yellow	1 cup	145	Trace	0.1	31	0.5	0	2	2 Starch
Instant, plain	1 packet	89	Trace	Tr	21	1.2	289	1 1/2	1 1/2 Starch

STARCH CHOICES

	Edible Portion	Cal	Fat (g)	Sat Fat (g)	Carb (g)	Fiber (g)	Sod. (mgs)	Carb Choices	Exchanges
Grains									
Arrowroot flour	3 Tbsp	80	0	0	20	0	0	1	1 Starch
Banana flour, commercial	3 Tbsp	81	0.4	0.2	21	0.4	1	1 1/2	1 1/2 Starch
Carob flour	1 cup	229	1	0.1	92	41	36	6	6 Starch
Cassava, fresh root, cooked	1/2 cup	110	0.2	0	27	1.3	9	2	2 Starch
Cornmeal, dry, whole grain	1 cup	442	4	0.6	94	8.9	43	6 1/2	6 1/2 Starch
Cornmeal, degermed, enriched	1 cup	505	2	0.3	107	10.2	4	7	6 Starch
Cornstarch	1 Tbsp	30	Trace	Tr	7	0.1	1	1/2	7 Starch
Eddo, dasheen, taro									
Fresh tuber, raw	1/2 cup	58	0.1	0	13.8	2.1	6	1	1 Starch
Tuber, cooked	1/2 cup	94	0	0	22.8	3.4	10	1 1/2	1/2 Starch
Tuber, fried	1/2 cup	164	5.7	1.5	27.7	4	198	198	2 Starch, 1 Fat
Plantain									
Green, fried slices	1/2 cup	134	6.6	0.9	20	1.5	4	1	Starch, 1 Fat
Plantain, cooked slices	1 cup	179	Trace	0.1	48	3.5	8	3	
Flour, commercial	3 Tbsp	71	0.2	0	19	0.3	0	1	1 Starch
Yam, yam pie									
Fresh root, raw	1/2 cup	89	0.1	0	21	0	7	1 1/2	1 1/2 Starch
Fresh root, cooked	1 small	95	0	0	21	0	7	1 1/2	1 1/2 Starch
Flour	3 Tbsp	74	0	0	18	0.4	0	1	1 Starch

STARCH CHOICES

	Edible Portion	Cal	Fat (g)	Sat Fat (g)	Carb (g)	Fiber (g)	Sod. (mgs)	Carb Choices	Exchanges
Starchy Vegetables									
Baked beans, pork and tomato sauce, canned	1/3 cup	76	0.8	0.3	15.2	3.2	355	1	1 Starch
Peas, black-eyed (crowder) cooked	1/2 cup	100	0.5	0.1	17.9	5.6	3	1	1 Starch + 1 lean meat
Sweet potato, baked with skin	1 potato	150	Trace	Tr	35	4.4	15	2	2 Starch
Sweet potato, boiled, no skin	1 potato	164	Trace	0.1	38	2.8	20	2 1/2	2 1/2 Starch
Sweet potato, candied	2 1/2" × 2" piece	144	3	1.4	29	2.5	74	2	2 Starch
Sweet potato, canned in syrup	1 cup	212	1	0.1	50	5.9	76	3	4 Starch

FRUIT CHOICES

	Edible Portion	Cal	Fat (g)	Sat Fat (g)	Carb (g)	Fiber (g)	Sod. (mgs)	Carb Choices	Exchanges
Ackee, fruit, raw	1/2 cup	180	17.5	0	5.5	0.3	Tr	1/2	3 fat, 1/2 fruit
Breadfruit	1 cup	227	0.51	0.10	60	10.8	4	4	4 Fruit
Carambola (starfruit), raw, whole	1 (3 5/8")	30	Trace	Tr	7	2.5	2	1/2	1/2 Fruit
Carambola (starfruit), raw, sliced	1 cup	36	Trace	Tr	8	2.9	2	1/2	1/2 Fruit
Cherry, West Indies									
Fruit, ripe	3 oz.	32	0.3	0	7.7	0.4	7	1/2	1/2 Fruit
Juice, fresh	1/3 cup	21	0.3	0	4.8	0.3	3	0	1/3 Fruit

FRUIT CHOICES

	Edible Portion	Cal	Fat (g)	Sat Fat (g)	Carb (g)	Fiber (g)	Sod. (mgs)	Carb Choices	Exchanges
Chocho, christophine, chayote									
Fruit, raw	1 each	38	0.3	0	9	3.5	4	1/2	1 Fruit
Fruit, cooked, drained	1/2 cup	19	0.4	0	4	2.2	1	0	1/3 Fruit
Custard apple	1/2 cup	114	0.7	0.3	28	2.7	5	2	2 Fruit
Governor plum	3 oz.	108	0	0	29.5	0.5	0	2	2 Fruit
Guana									
Whole	3 oz.	51	0.6	0.2	11.9	5.6	3	1	1 Fruit
Pulp only	1/2 cup	42	0.5	0.1	9.8	4.5	2	1/2	1 Fruit
Nectar	4 fluid oz.	72	0.1	0	18	1.8	0	1	1 1/4 Fruit
Guinep, genip	3 oz.	59	0.2	0	19.9	1.4	0	1	1 1/4 Fruit
Hog plum	3 oz.	70	2.1	0	13.8	1	0	1	1 Fruit
Jackfruit	1/2 cup	78	0.3	0	19.8	1.3	2	1	1/3 Fruit
Japanese plum (loquat, mayapple), fresh	3/4 cup cubed	53	0.2	0	13.6	1.9	1	1	1 Fruit
Java plum	1 cup	60	0.2	0	15.6	0.3	14	1	1 1/2 Fruit
Jujube	3 oz.	79	0.2	0	20.2	1.4	3	1	1 Fruit
Mammee apple	1/4	51	0.5	0	12.5	1	15	1	2 Fruit
Mango raw, whole	1 mango	135	1	0.1	35	3.7	4	2	2 Fruit
Mango. raw. sliced	1 cup	107	Trace	0.1	28	3	3	2	2 Fruit
Mangosteen, canned, drained	1/2 cup	76	0.8	0	18.6	1.3	0	1	1 Fruit
Paw paw, papaya									
Fresh fruit	1/2 medium	59	0.2	0	14.9	2.7	5	1	1 Fruit
Nectar, canned	4 fluid oz.	71	0.2	0	18	0.8	6	1	1 1/3 Fruit
Permimmon, Japanese, soft, fresh	1/2 fruit (2 ½" diameter)	59	0.2	0	15.6	3	1	1	1 Fruit

FRUIT CHOICES

	Edible Portion	Cal	Fat (g)	Sat Fat (g)	Carb (g)	Fiber (g)	Sod. (mgs)	Carb Choices	Exchanges
Plantain, raw, without peel	1 medium	218	1	0.3	57	4.1	7	4	3 Starch
Rose apple	3 oz.	25	0.3	0	5.7	1.1	0	1/2	1/2 Fruit
Sapodilla, naseberry	1/2 cup	100	1.3	0.2	224	6.4	14	1 1/2	1 1/2 Fruit
Sorrel									
Raw	3 oz.	55	1	0	12	1	0	1	1 Fruit
Dried	1 oz.	304	2.6	0	74.1	12	0	5	1 1/2 Fruit
Soursop	1/4 fruit	103	0.5	0	26.3	5.1	22	2	1 3/4 Fruit
Surinam cherry	1 cup	33	0.4	0	7.5	0.6	3	1/2	1 Fruit
Sweetsop, sugar apple	1 fruit	96	0.2	0	24.6	1.6	1	1 1/2	1 1/2 Fruit
Watermelon, fresh	1 1/2 cup	57	0.3	0	14.3	0.8	2	1	1 Fruit

VEGETABLE CHOICES

	Edible Portion	Cal	Fat (g)	Sat Fat (g)	Carb (g)	Fiber (g)	Sod. (mgs)	Carb Choices	Exchanges
Callaloo, cooked	1/2 cup	19	0.2	0	3.7	1.2	19	0	1/2 Veg
Collards, cooked, from raw	1 cup	49	1	0.1	9	5.3	17	1/2	2 Veg
Collards, cooked, from frozen	1 cup	61	1	0.1	12	4.8	85	1	2 Veg
Dandelion greens, cooked	1 cup	35	1	0.2	7	3	46	1/2	2 Veg
Kale, cooked, from raw	1 cup	36	1	0.1	7	2.6	30	1/2	2 Veg
Kale, cooked, from frozen	1 cup	39	1	0.1	7	2.6	20	1/2	2 Veg
Mirliton (vegetable pear), cooked	1/2 cup	19	0.4	0.1	4.1	2.2	1	0	1 Veg

VEGETABLE CHOICES

	Edible Portion	Cal	Fat (g)	Sat Fat (g)	Carb (g)	Fiber (g)	Sod. (mgs)	Carb Choices	Exchanges
Mustard greens, cooked	1 cup	21	Trace	Tr	3	2.8	22	0	2 Veg
Okra, cooked from raw	1 cup	51	Trace	0.1	12	4	8	1	2 Veg
Okra, cooked from frozen	1 cup	52	1	0.1	11	5.2	6	1	2 Veg
Oyster mushroom, raw	1/2 large	32	0.3	0	4.8	1.7	13	0	1 Veg
Turnip, cooked	1 cup	33	Trace	Tr	8	3.1	78	1/2	2 Veg
Turnip greens, cooked from raw	1 cup	29	Trace	0.1	6	5	42	1/2	2 Veg
Turnip greens, cooked from frozen	1 cup	49	1	0.2	8	5.6	25	1/2	2 Veg

MILK CHOICES

	Edible Portion	Cal	Fat (g)	Sat Fat (g)	Carb (g)	Fiber (g)	Sod. (mgs)	Carb Choices	Exchanges
Other Milk									
Buffalo's milk, whole	8 fluid oz.	237	17	11.2	12.7	0	127	1	1 milk, 2 fat
Goat's milk, whole	8 fluid oz.	168	10	6.6	11	0	122	1	1 milk, 1 fat
Sheep's milk, whole	8 fluid oz.	264	17	11.2	13	0	107	1	1 milk, 2 fat

Fish, Poultry, and Meat Choices

	Edible Portion	Cal	Fat (g)	Sat Fat (g)	Carb (g)	Fiber (g)	Sod. (mgs)	Carb Choices	Exchanges
Amberjack									
Raw	1 oz.	24	0.3	0	0	0	0	0	1 Very Lean Meat
Dried	1 oz.	76	1.3	0	0	0	0	0	1 Very Lean Meat
Anchovy	1 oz.	24	0.3	0	0	0	0	0	1 Very Lean Meat
Barracuda	1 oz.	31	0.7	0	0	0	0	0	1 Very Lean Meat
Bonito	1 oz.	47	2	0	0	0	0	0	1 Very Lean Meat
Butterfish									
Raw	1 oz.	41	2.2	0	0	0	25	0	1 Very Lean Meat
Baked	1 oz.	52	2.9	0	0	0	32	0	1 Very Lean Meat
Carp, common	1 oz.	35	1.6	0.3	0	0	14	0	1 Very Lean Meat
Catfish, breaded, fried	1 oz.	65	4	1	2	0.2	79	0	1 Medium-Fat Meat
Crawfish	1 oz.	19	0.26	0.04	0	0	17	0	1 Very Lean Meat
Croaker, cooked	1 oz.	37	0.9	0	0	0	33	0	1 Very Lean Meat
Croaker, raw	1 oz.	29	0.9	0.3	0	0	24	0	1 Very Lean Meat
Jacks	1 oz.	28	0.4	0	0	0	0	0	1 Very Lean Meat
Kingfish	1 oz.	29	0.8	0	0	0	23	0	1 Very Lean Meat
Porgy	1 oz.	31	0.9	0	0	0	0	0	1 Very Lean Meat

FISH, POULTRY, and MEAT CHOICES

	Edible Portion	Cal	Fat (g)	Sat Fat (g)	Carb (g)	Fiber (g)	Sod. (mgs)	Carb Choices	Exchanges
Snapper	1 oz.	25	0.2	0	0	0	19	0	1 Very Lean Meat
Turtle									
Raw	1 oz.	25	0.1	0	0	0	0	0	1 Very Lean Meat
Canned	1 oz.	29	0.2	0	0	0	0	0	1 Very Lean Meat
Whiting, "Banga Mary"	1 oz.	26	0.1	0	0	0	0	0	1 Lean Meat
Offals									
Brain, beef, raw	1 oz.	35	2.6	0.6	0	0	29	0	1 Medium-Fat Meat
Feet, trotters									
Pork, medium fat	1 oz.	79	6	0	0	0	0	0	1 Very Lean Meat
Heart									
Beef	1 oz.	33	1	0.3	0.4	0	18	0	1 Very Lean Meat
Mutton or lamb	1 oz.	34	1.6	0.6	0	0	25	0	1 Very Lean Meat
Pork	1 oz.	33	1.2	0.3	0.1	0	16	0	1 Lean Meat
Hogshead cheese (head cheese, jellied pork)	1 oz.	45	3.1	0	0	0	236	0	1 Very Lean Meat
Intestine or tripe									
Beef	1 oz.	27	1.1	0.5	0	0	13	0	1 Lean Meat
Pork	1 oz.	44	2.6	0	0	0	14	0	1 Very Lean Meat

Fish, Poultry, and Meat Choices

	Edible Portion	Cal	Fat (g)	Sat Fat (g)	Carb (g)	Fiber (g)	Sod. (mgs)	Carb Choices	Exchanges
Kidney									
Beef	1 oz.	30	1	0.3	0.6	0	50	0	1 Very Lean Meat
Mutton or lamb	1 oz.	27	1	0.3	0.2	0	43	0	1 Very Lean Meat
Pork	1 oz.	28	1	0.3	0	0	34	0	1 Very Lean Meat
Liver									
Beef, raw	1 oz.	40	1	0.4	1.6	0	20	0	1 Very Lean Meat
Beef, stewed	1 oz.	45	1.4	0.5	1	0	19	0	1 Very Lean Meat
Chicken, raw	1 oz.	38	1.8	0.5	0.2	0	24	0	1 Very Lean Meat
Mutton or lamb, raw	1 oz.	39	1.4	0.5	0.5	0	19	0	1 Very Lean Meat
Pork, raw	1 oz.	37	1	0.3	0.7	0	24	0	1 Very Lean Meat
Pork, cooked	1 oz.	46	1.2	0.4	1	0	14	0	1 Very Lean Meat
Lung									
Beef	1 oz.	26	0.7	0.3	0	0	55	0	1 Very Lean Meat
Mutton or lamb	1 oz.	26	0.7	0	0	0	44	0	1 Very Lean Meat
Pork	1 oz.	24	0.8	0.3	0	0	43	0	1 Very Lean Meat
Tail									
Ox, leanonly, raw	1 oz.	48	2.8	0	0	0	31	0	1 Lean Meat
Stewed (salt added)	1 oz.	68	3.7	0	0	0	53	0	1 Lean Meat

Fish, Poultry, and Meat Choices

	Edible Portion	Cal	Fat (g)	Sat Fat (g)	Carb (g)	Fiber (g)	Sod. (mgs)	Carb Choices	Exchanges
Pig, in brine	1 oz.	119	11.6	0	0	0	0	0	1 High-fat Meat, 1/2 Fat
Pig, fresh	1 oz.	105	9.3	3.2	0	0	0	0	1 High-fat Meat
Pork trotters and tails, salted/ boiled	1 oz.	78	6.2	0	0	0	449	0	1 Medium-fat Meat
Tongue									
Beef, fresh, raw	1 oz.	62	4.5	1.9	1	0	19	0	1 Medium-fat Meat
Pickled, boiled (fat and skin removed)	1 oz.	81	6.6	0	0	0	278	0	1 Medium-fat Meat
Mutton or lamb, fresh, raw	1 oz.	62	4.8	1.8	0	0	22	0	1 Medium-fat Meat
Pork, fresh, raw	1 oz.	63	4.8	1.6	0	0	31	0	1 Medium-fat Meat
Black pudding, fried	1 oz.	85	6	2.4	0	0	336	0	1 Medium-fat Meat
Other meats: Game									
Goat, raw	1 oz.	30	0.6	0	0	0	0	0	1 Very Lean Meat
Mammals, dressed	1 oz.	34	1	0	0	0	0	0	1 Very Lean Meat
Birds, dressed	1 oz.	40	1.4	0	0	0	0	0	1 Very Lean Meat
Guinea pig, flesh only	1 oz.	27	0.4	0	0	0	0	0	1 Very Lean Meat
Iguana	1 oz.	31	0	0	0	0	0	0	1 Very Lean Meat

Fish, Poultry, and Meat Choices

	Edible Portion	Cal	Fat (g)	Sat Fat (g)	Carb (g)	Fiber (g)	Sod. (mgs)	Carb Choices	Exchanges
Rabbit, flesh, raw	1 oz.	38	1.5	0.2	0	0	11	0	1 Very Lean Meat
Rabbit, flesh, stewed	1 oz.	50	2.1	0	0	0	0	0	1 Very Lean Meat

Fat Choices

	Edible Portion	Cal	Fat (g)	Sat Fat (g)	Carb (g)	Fiber (g)	Sod. (mgs)	Carb Choices	Exchanges
Chitterlings, boiled	2 Tbsp.	37	3.3	1.5	0	0	3	0	1 Fat
Cracklings, pork (gratons), cooked	1 1/2 Tbsp.	46	3.6	1.2	0.1	0	198	0	1 Fat
Salt pork, cooked	1/4 oz.	51	5.4	1.9	0	0	91	0	1 Fat

Resources

American Association of Diabetes Educators (AADE)

800–338–3633 or 312–424–2426

Diabetes Educator Access Line: 1–800–TEAMUP4 (1–800–832–6874)

www.diabeteseducator.org

A group of more than 10,000 health professionals dedicated to advocating quality diabetes education and care.

American Diabetes Association (ADA)

800–DIABETES (1–800–342–2383)—National Call Center has a trained staff that answers calls and e-mails from people with diabetes.

www.diabetes.org

With a mission to prevent and cure diabetes, the ADA publishes many books and resources for people with diabetes, including *Diabetes Forecast*, a monthly magazine.

American Dietetic Association (ADA)

800–877–1600

www.eatright.org

To promote optimal nutrition and well-being, ADA publishes many books and other resources for consumers and professionals. On the website, click on "Find a Nutrition Professional" to find a dietitian near you.

Consumer Nutrition Hotline, a toll-free call center that provides a referral service to registered dietitians. 800–877–1600

Association of Black Psychologists (ABPsi)

202–722–0808

www.abpsi.org

African-American mental health professional who work toward "the liberation of the African Mind, empowerment of the African Character, and enlivement and illumination of the African Spirit."

Materials: ABPsi's Website has a Black Psychologist directory that provides patients with the names and locations of African American psychologist in their area.

Centers for Disease Control and Prevention (CDC)
National Center for Chronic Disease Prevention and Health Promotion
Division of Diabetes Translation
800–CDC–INFO (800–232–4636) or 770–448–5000
www.cdc.gov/diabetes
The CDC distributes several publications including a patient guide for people with diabetes (in English and Spanish). Supports state-based diabetes programs that develop and maintain local programs. Internet home page includes fact sheets, statistics, publications, and information about state diabetes prevention and control programs.

dLife: The Diabetes Health Company
866–354–3366 or 203–454–6985
www.dlife.com
Offers a variety of resources to empower people with diabetes and support their emotional, motivational, and practical needs. Provides information and community support through television programs, online forums, and mobile and e-mail outreach.

National Diabetes Education Program (NDEP)
800–438–5383
www.ndep.nih.gov
Offers diabetes education materials (free or at little cost) toward improving the treatment and outcomes for people with diabetes, promoting early diagnosis, and preventing or delaying the onset of diabetes.

National Institute of Diabetes and Digestive and Kidney Diseases (NIDDK)
www.niddk.nih.gov
Part of the National Institutes of Health, NIDDK is the government's lead agency for diabetes research. The NIDDK operates three diabetes information clearinghouses and funds six diabetes research and training centers and eight diabetes endocrinology research centers.

National Medical Association (NMA)
202–347–1895
www.nmanet.org
Promotes health and wellness, eliminate health disparities in the African American community and supports physicians of color. The NMA website has a physician locator service to help you find a NMA-member doctor in your community.

Office of Minority Health Resource Center (OMH-RC)
800–444–6472
www.omhrc.gov
The largest resource and referral service on minority health in the nation offers information, publications, mailing lists, database searches, referrals, and more for African American and other people of color.

INDEX

About the Authors

Constance Brown-Riggs, MSEd, RD, CDE, CDN, an award winning registered dietitian, certified diabetes educator and national spokesperson for the American Dietetic Association, is the author of *Eating Soulfully and Healthfully with Diabetes* (iUniverse, 2006) and creator of the *Diabetes Soul Food Pyramid* (© 2001 CBR Nutrition Enterprises).

During her career, she has established herself as an expert on the subject of nutrition, diabetes, and the cultural issues that impact the health and healthcare of people of color. Her ability to translate her extensive academic and clinical knowledge of medical nutrition into clear, understandable terms have made her a nationally respected and much sought-after speaker, educator, and author. Her work has appeared in books for health professionals and healthcare consumers, and she has been a featured expert in national magazines such as *Essence*, *Real Health*, and *Diabetic Cooking*.

Through her active nutrition counseling practice in New York, she sees hundreds of individual patients. She also conducts diabetes education workshops and seminars—for schools, churches, and other organizations—which reach thousands of people each year.

She is past president of both the 5,000-member New York State Dietetic Association and of the Long Island Dietetic Association, a 500-member organization. And she is currently a national spokesperson with a specialty in African-American Nutrition for the American Dietetic Association. Her professional honors include 2009 Distinguished Dietitian Award from the New York State Dietetic Association and 2007 Diabetes Educator of the Year from the American Dietetic Association Diabetes Care and Education Practice Group.

She is passionate about creating opportunities to spread the word about health and nutrition, and developing educational tools which shorten the cultural distance between patients and caregivers. Every aspect of her work supports that mission. Learn more about her work at eatingsoulfully.com.

Tamara Jeffries, the former executive editor of *Essence* magazine, is a long-time health and wellness writer. Formerly the editor of *HealthQuest: The Publication of Black Wellness* and a contributing editor at *Health,* she has written articles for *Redbook*, *Parenting*, *Heart & Soul*, *Real Healt*, and other national publications as well as contributed to several health-related books. A 2009 recipient of the Rosalyn Carter Mental Health Journalism Fellowship, she currently teaches journalism at Bennett College for Women in North Carolina. Visit her Website at *www.TamaraJeffries.com.*